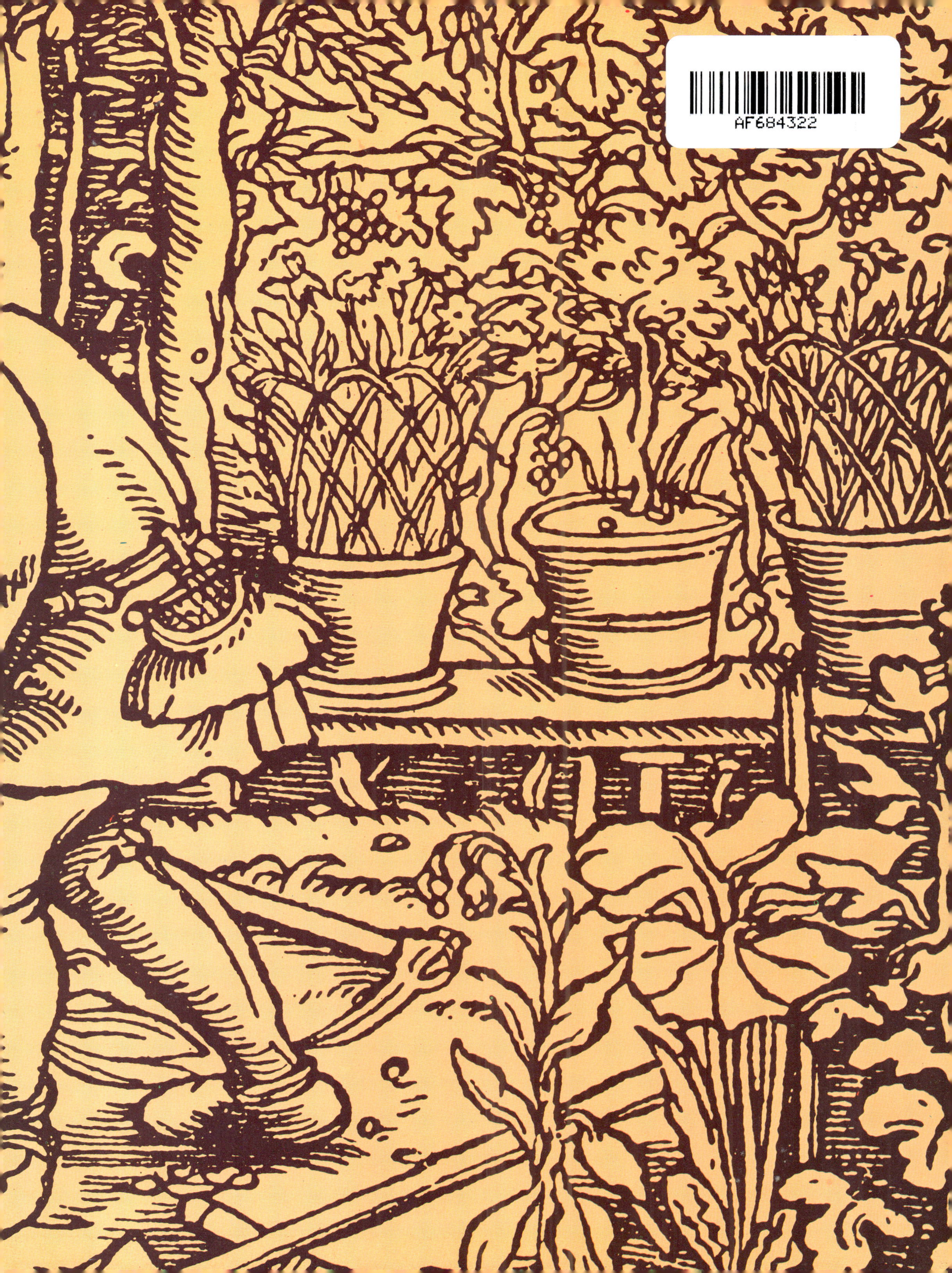

Folk Medicine Fact and Fiction

Frances Kennett

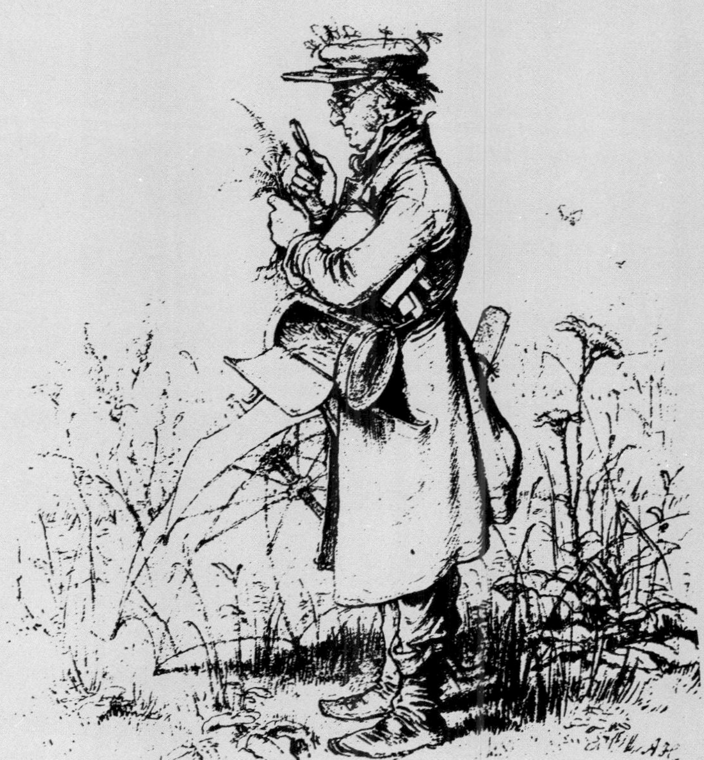

Marshall Cavendish

Picture credits.
Bibliotheque de l'Arsenal/R. Lalance: 16TR;
Bibliotheque Nationale/J. Gallus/Giraudon: 54;
Bodleian Library Oxford: MS Ashmole: 20BR; 36B; 12th Century Herbal: 26T; 13th Century Herbal: 26B; 68; 15th Century Herbal: 25; Gerards' Herbal 1597: 27;
courtesy British Epilepsy Association: 76R;
British Museum: 'Ague & Fever' Thomas Rowlandson: 33TL;
British Museum/courtesy Aldus Books: 34T; 55TR;
Camera Press: 44/5;
Roger Charity: 21B; 22BR;
Culpepper Ltd.: 17B;
C. M. Dixon: 9BR;
Dover Press: 'Handbook of Plants & Floral Ornament from Early Herbals': 18B; 48TL & TR; 49BC; 55BL; 62R;
'Early American Advertising Art': 35T;
'French Advertising Art': 81CR; 83L; 84TL; 85BR; 86CL;
Alan Duns: 21T;
Mary Evans Picture Library: 1; 3B; 10/11; 12T; 14TR; 17TL & TR; 19TL; 22TR & BL; 24TL & CR; 28; 31T; 34B; 40BL; 43BR; 46; 47TR & CR; 49T; BL & BR; 57BL; 59L; 64TL; 66CR; 67R; 69T; 70CR; 71; 72BL; 74TL; 78; 82; 87;
courtesy Mrs. E. L. Freud: 45;
John Garret: 39;
Gilcrease Institute of American History Oklahoma: 'Idols of Mandans' Karl Bodmer: 11B;
Graffiti: 30; 50;
Hahnemann House Museum: 40TL; 42CT;
Graeme Harris: 14B;
Heinneman Medical Books: 83TR & BR; 84BL;
Michael Holford: 9BL; 10BL; 14TL;
Brian Lake Books: 57TR; 63; 79R;
courtesy Dr. Felix Mann/Anton Last: 38;
Mansell Collection: Endpapers: 6/7; 12B; 13; 15; 16B; 17C; 18T; 23B; 24CL; 32; 35B; 42L; 47TL & BL; 52; 53TR; 58; 59BR; 60; 61; 64BR; 65R; 66BL; 67L; 70TL; 73; 75; 76L; 77CR; 81;
Arboria Mella: 29;
National Gallery of Scotland: 23T;
Gerald Nason: 8;
Pharmaceutical Society of Great Britain: 47CB; 48BC; & BR;
Graham Percy: 20T;
Roger Philips: cover;
Harry Price Library: 10TC; 11T;
Putti Collection/Rizzoli Institute: 31B;
Arthur Rackham: 9C; 20BL;
Radio Times Hulton Picture Library: 19TR; 24B; 33TR; 36T; 42/3; 53BL; 72TL; 85BL; 86TR;
Sue Richards: 65L; 66TL; 69B; 72TR; 79L;
courtesy Royal College of Surgeons: 62L;
Royal Photographic Society: 37;
Scala: 19B; 40/1T;
G. D. Searle & Co. Ltd.: 80;
Tate Gallery: 'The Fairy Feller's Master Stroke' Richard Dadd: 2/3;
Patrick Thurston: 4/5; 40/1B; 41R;
Transworld Feature Syndicate: 16TL;
courtesy Wellcome Trustees: 18R; 33B; 56; 81BL; 84BR; 85TL;

Editor Yvonne Deutch

Designer Chris Lower

Picture Researcher Sheila Thompson

Published by
Marshall Cavendish Books Limited
58 Old Compton Street
London W1V 5PA

ISBN 0 85685 162 0

Printed and bound in Italy by New Interlitho SpA.

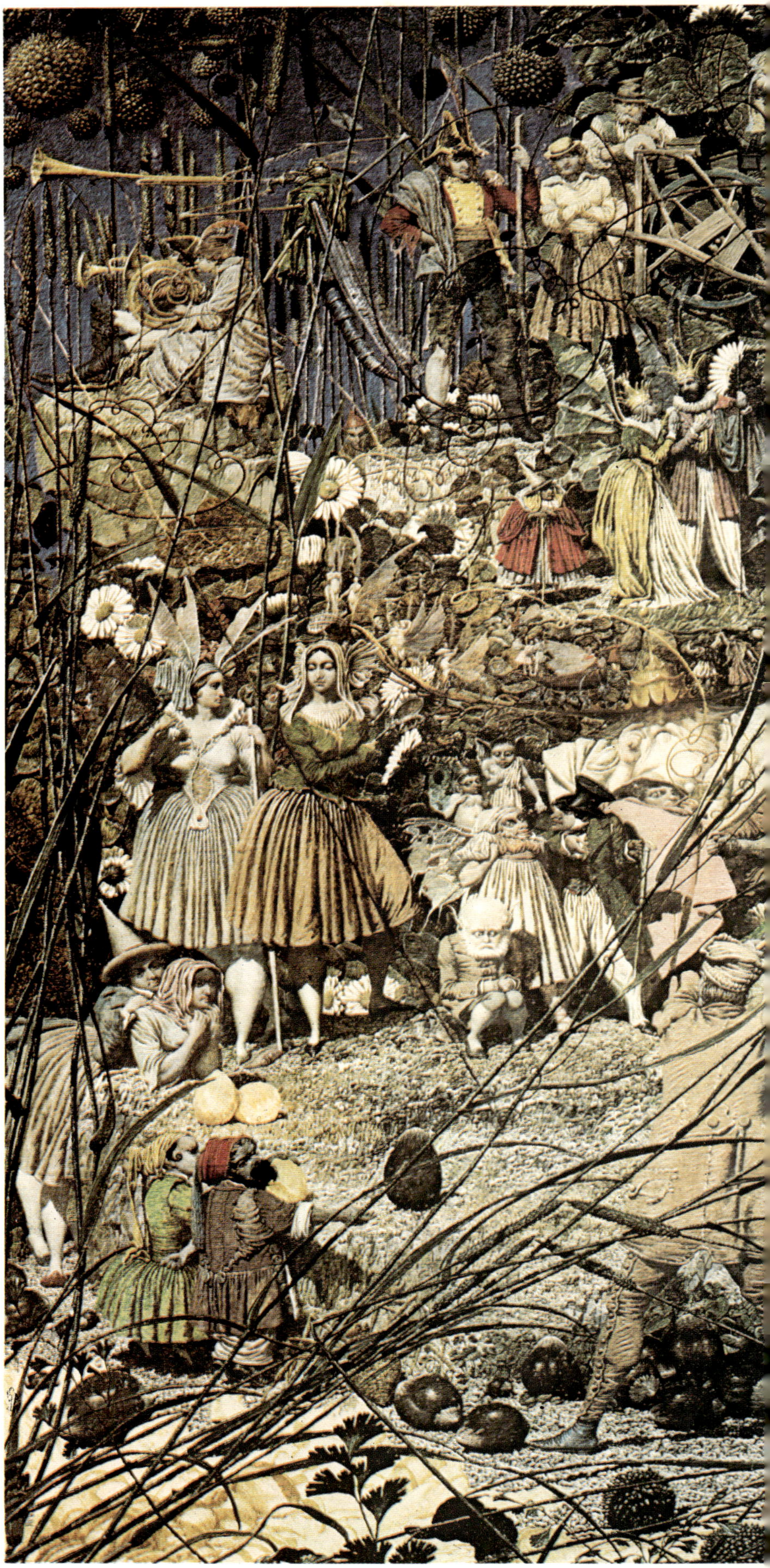

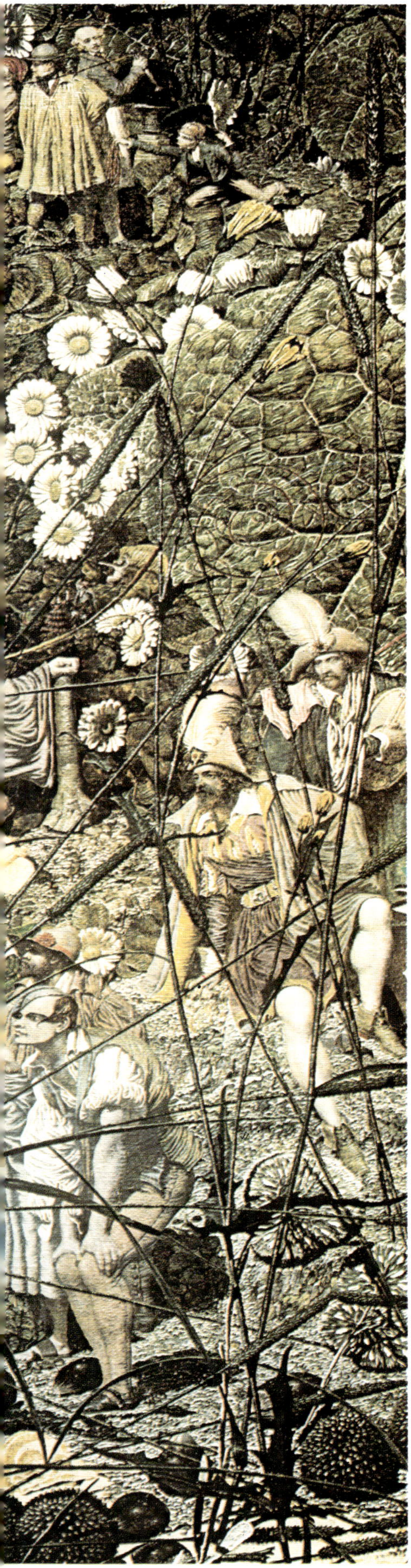

Introduction

As modern medicine becomes more impersonal, people are recalling with some wistfulness old country cures administered by parents and grandparents over the generations. A soothing mixture of honey and lemon for a cough, cool green dock leaves to take away the sting of a nettle, delicious herb teas and brews for upset tummies – these common treatments are part of an intriguing body of knowledge which has existed side by side with professional medicine through the centuries. *Folk Medicine: Fact and Fiction* explores the ideas and basic theories behind folk medicine, shows how quack medicine exploited many of its remedies, and how, nowadays, fringe medicine is carrying on many of its traditions.

The author, Frances Kennett, has shrewdly separated fact from fable in her account – for although some of the cures have worked over the years, many are based on little more than ignorance and old wives' tales. But whether they work or not, the remedies are fascinating in themselves. All of them are of interest to people who want to go back to a natural way of health, and to anyone curious about superstitions which are still prevalent today. Folk medicine is not concerned only with illness – there is an extensive section on childbirth, as well as a selection of beauty treatments for hair and skin which can be made up at home. Illustrated with beautiful and unusual pictures, *Folk Medicine: Fact and Fiction* provides entertaining reading, as well as returning you to a rich and valuable heritage of practical folklore.

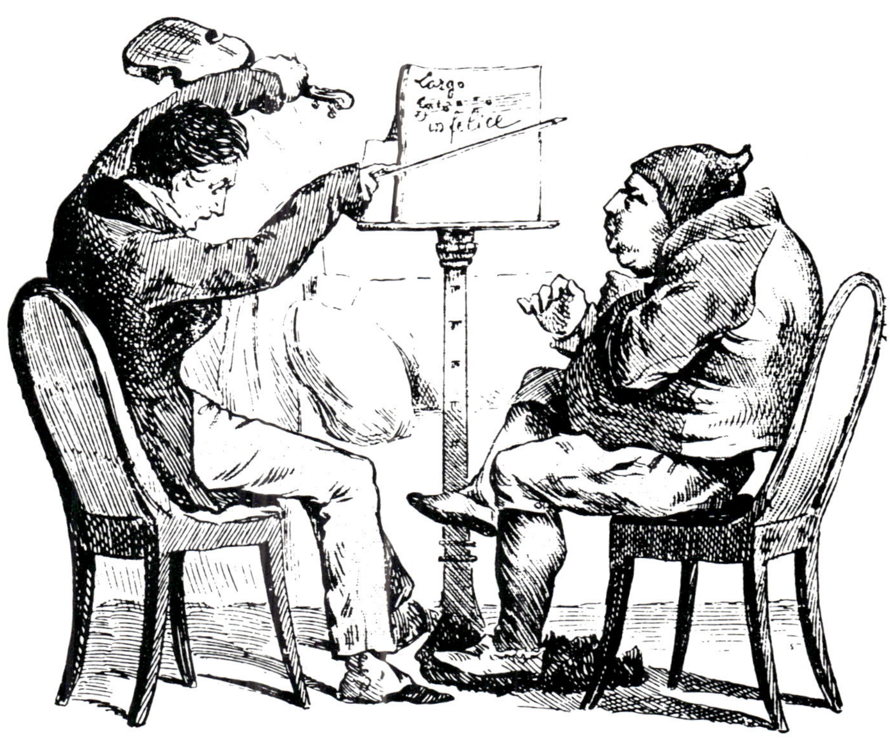

Contents

Folk medicine through the ages

Remedies and cures

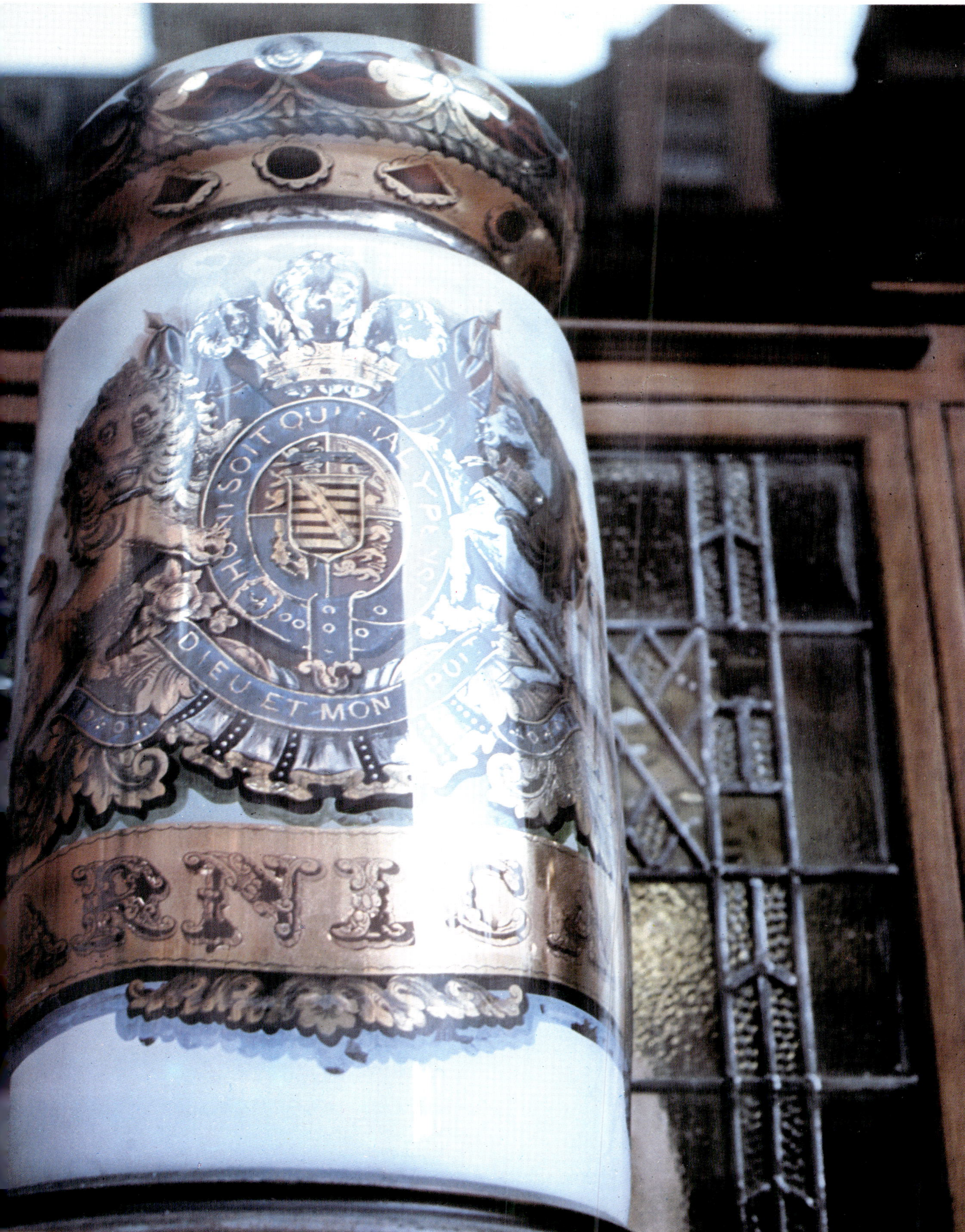
SOIT QUI MAL Y PENSE
DIEU ET MON

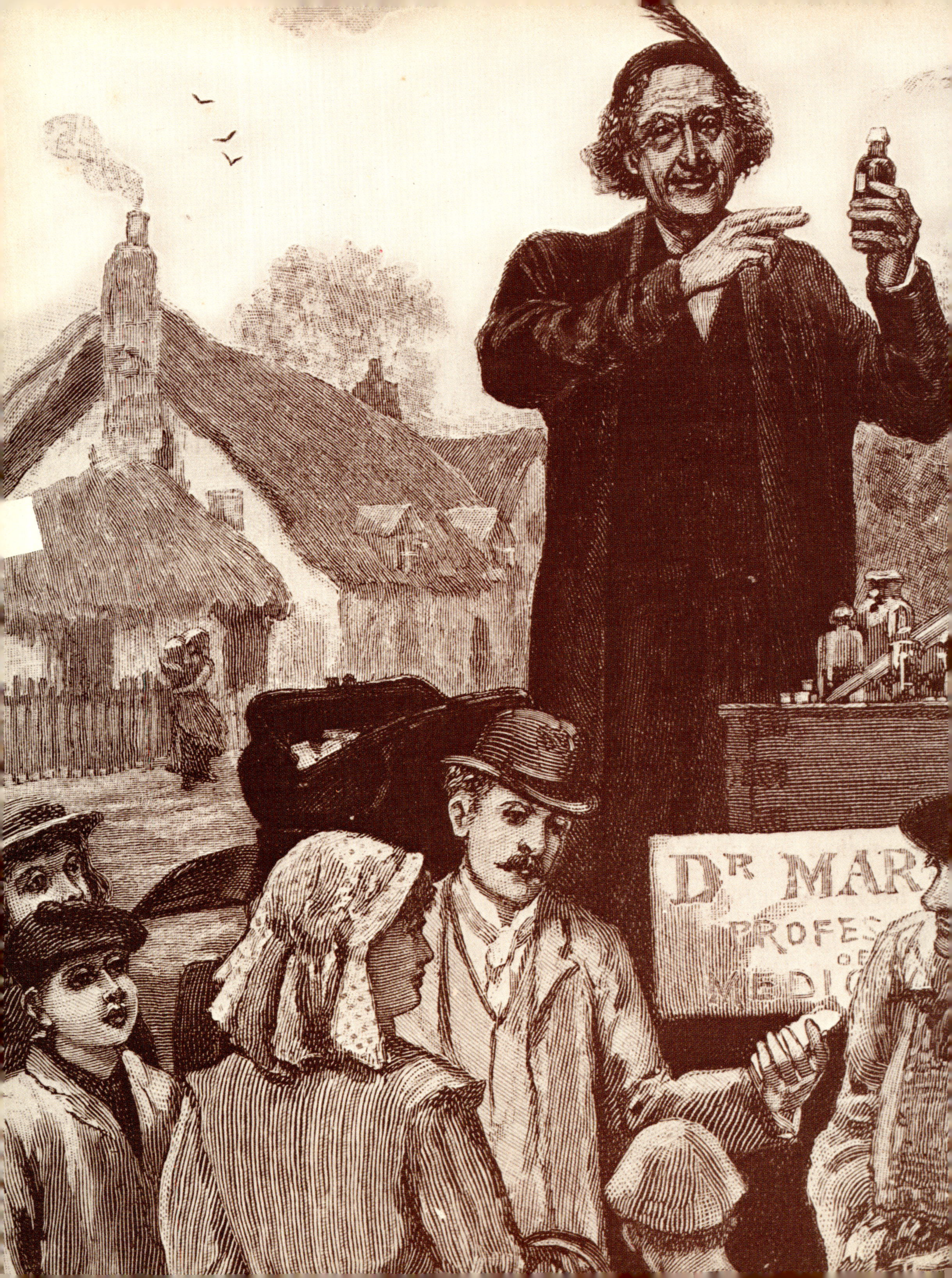

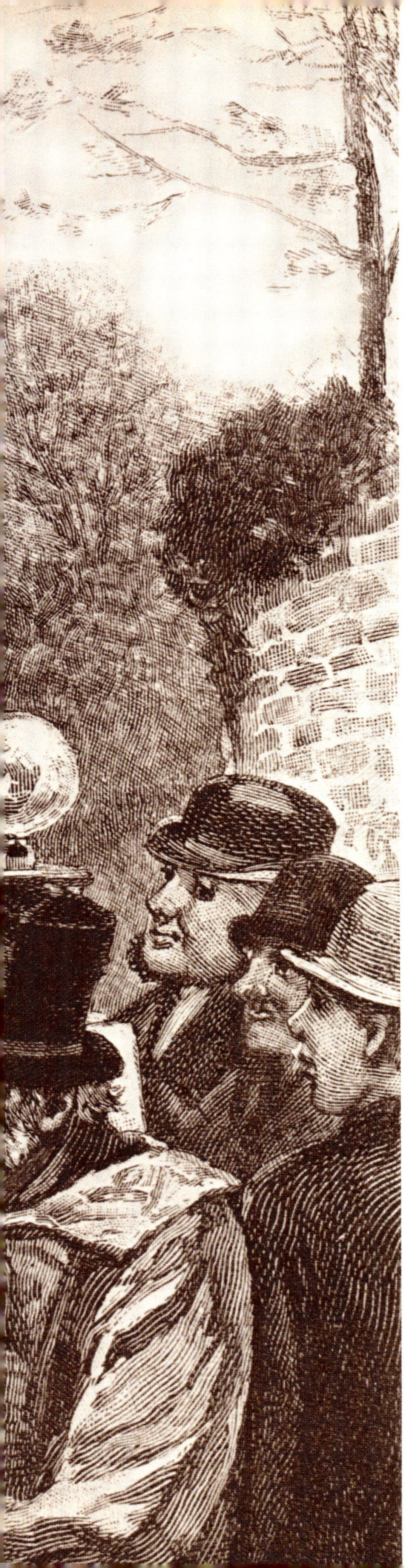

Folk Medicine Through the Ages

A quack doctor selling his wares. Many patent remedies were derived from folk medicine and claimed as new inventions.

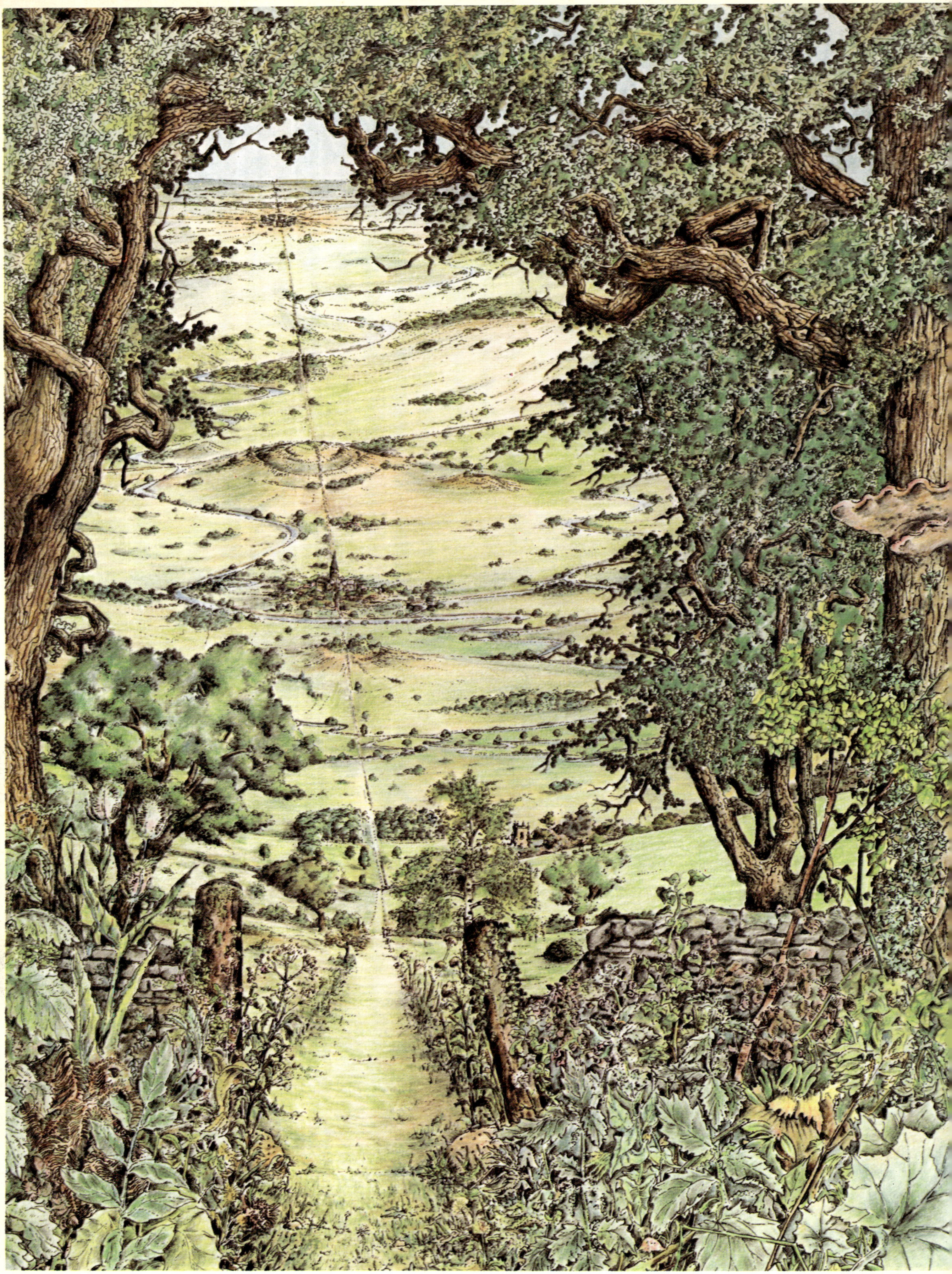

Folk medicine

'Folk medicine' is a very general term, covering a wide variety of medical, traditional or superstitious practices. All of them have certain features in common, which help to explain why they have survived so long, and why people have accepted them through the ages. The origins of folk medicine obviously link up with other significant areas of man's experience, such as his god-worship, or his understanding of the forces of nature. It has naturally inherited many magical elements from such a background, and effective cures are typically assumed to have non-rational explanations.

This apparent lack of cause is one of the major features of many folk remedies, and is both a strength and a weakness – the first because everyone loves a mystery, and is very ready to believe in a miraculous success; the second, because many people go on doing things to their bodies because they have faith in the ritual itself, without acknowledging scientific evidence that the process is dangerous. This book attempts to explain some of the traditions of folk medicine, analyzes its virtues, examines its failings, and reveals some of the ways in which modern doctors are beginning to learn from this traditional art.

Extreme left *The earth abounds with natural sources of healing. Here the artist has depicted 'ley' lines which link up magically significant areas of the landscape. Earth and fertility deities are common to all cultures.* **Middle** *An Indian tree goddess.* **Above right** *Puck, or Robin Goodfellow, was traditionally known as a mischief-making fairy. This illustration is by Arthur Rackham from Shakespeare's* A Midsummer Night's Dream. **Below right** *The god Pan represented the violent side of nature, as well as its fertile aspects. This lovely illustration of the deity is from a sixteenth-century Italian dish, delicately coloured.*

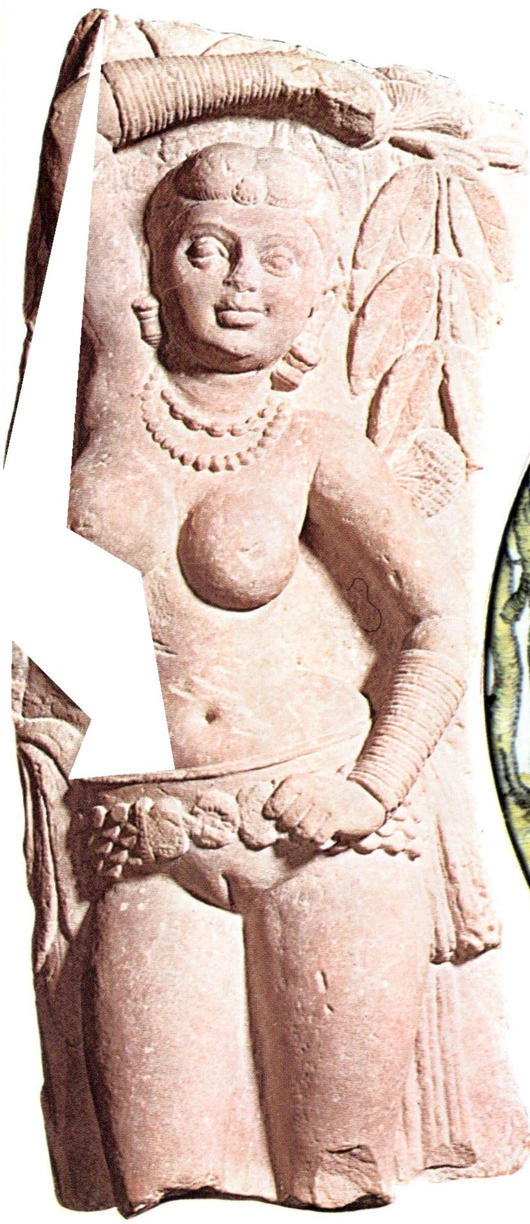

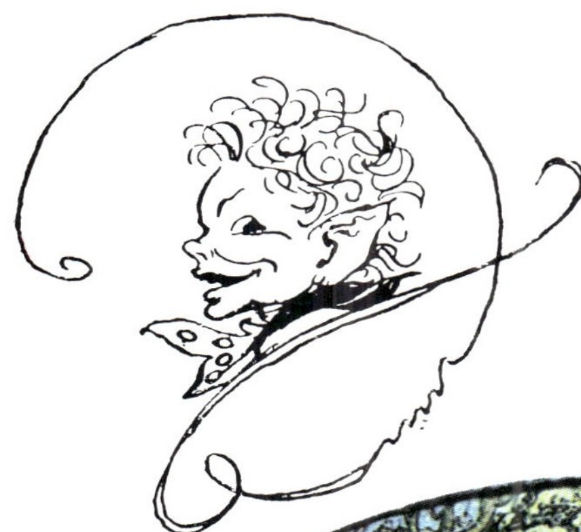

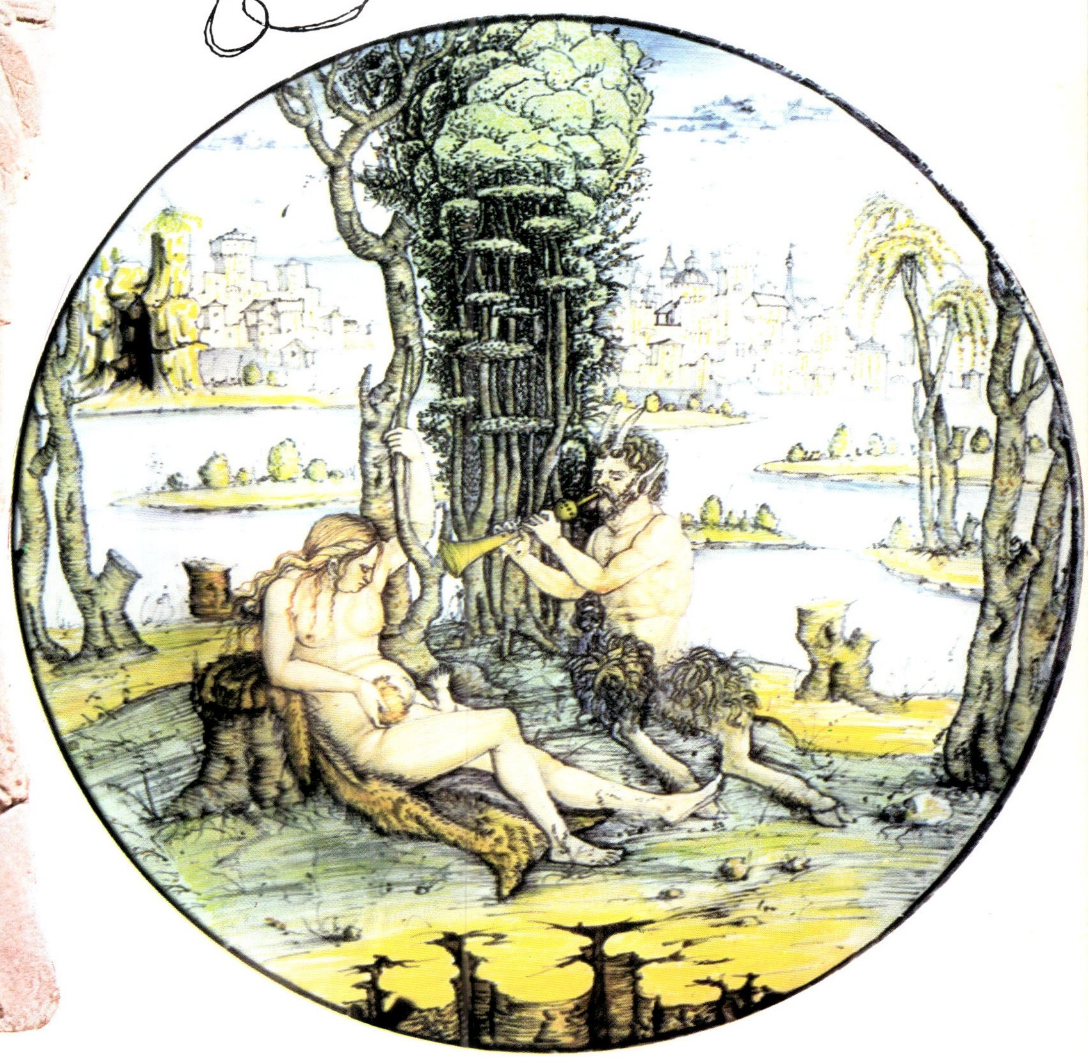

Primitive theories of illness attributed disease to the presence of demonic beings. **Above** *and* **below** *(centre) Witch doctors were specialists in curing ailments by their ability to eject demons.* **Right** *The demons Asmodeus (above) and Astaroth (below).* **Below left** *In order to gain unusual powers many rituals were enacted to mimic the desired skill. This Indian 'bird man' mimics flight in his ritual dance.*

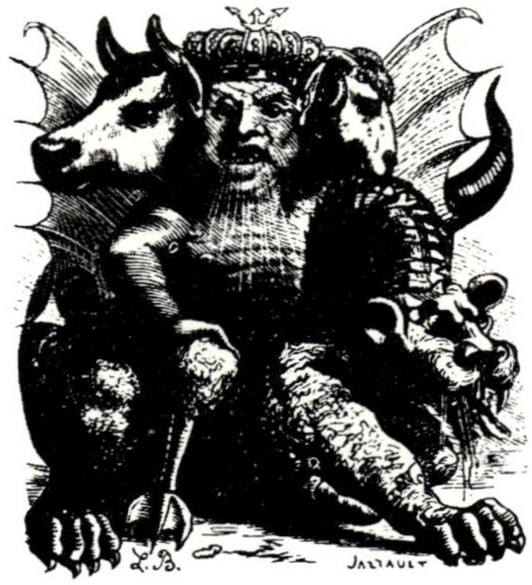

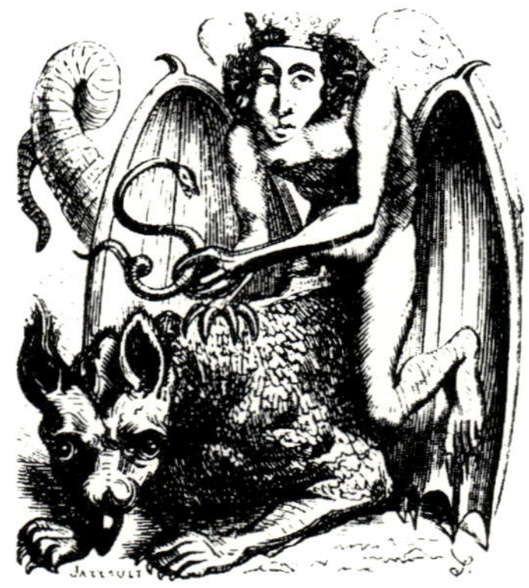

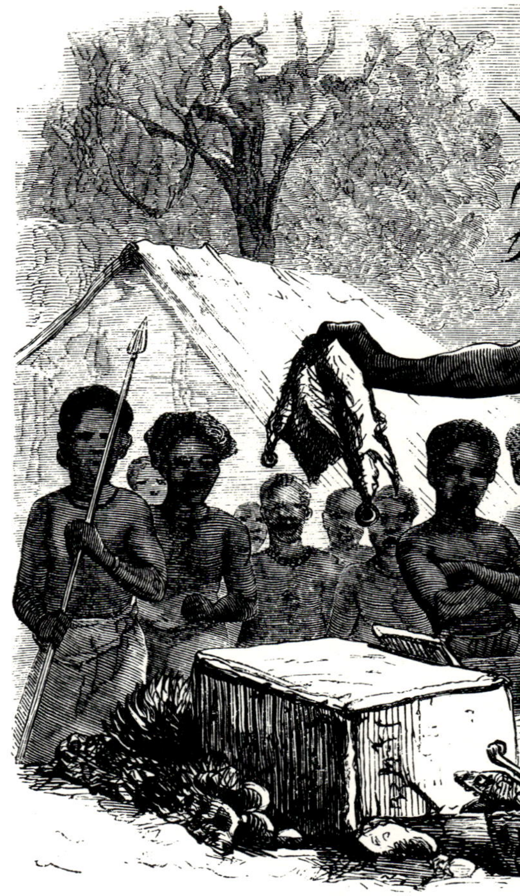

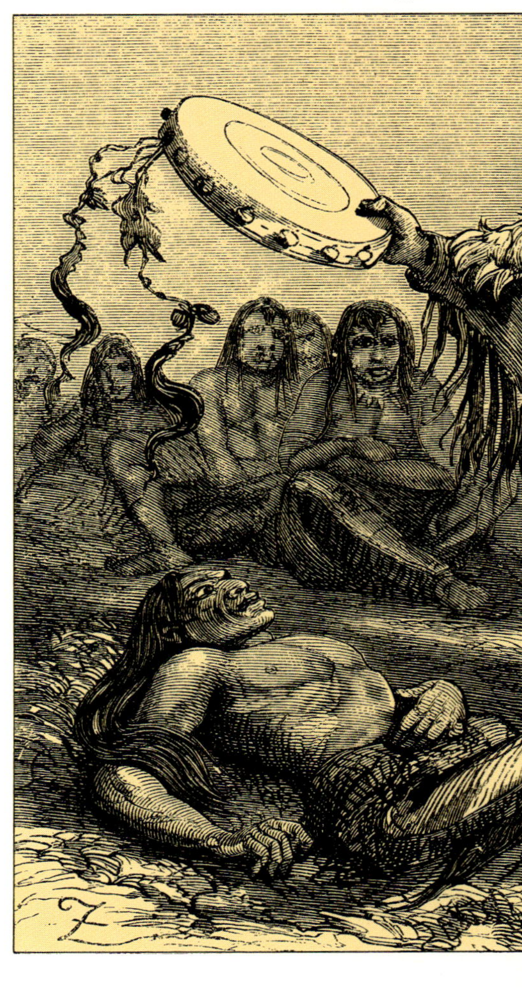

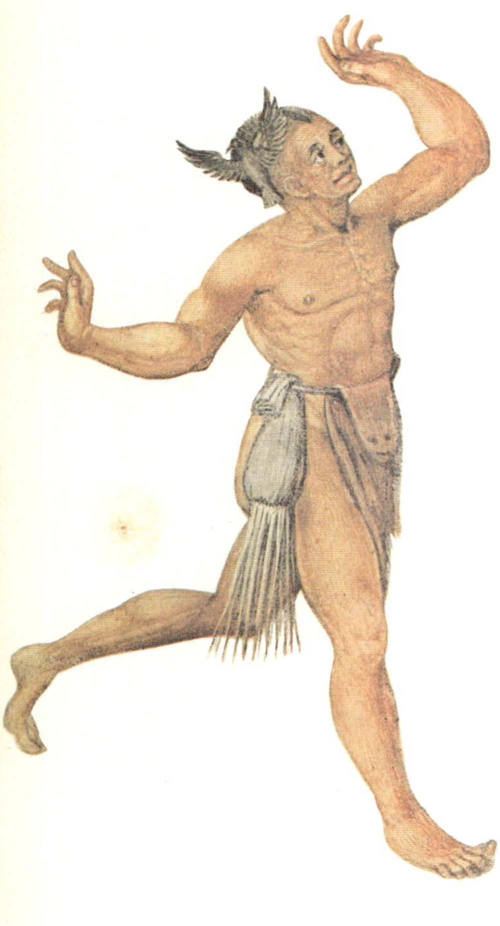

Medicine and the Devil

The very earliest explanations for bodily ills tended to put the blame on the gods. Most illnesses of a serious nature seem to arrive out of the blue, and pass from person to person in an unseen, mysterious way. It seemed logical to primitive man that the spirits who controlled the other great forces of the world, the wind, rain, sun, moon, the seas and rivers, must also be responsible for these dreadful visitations on the human race.

In some societies, diseases of all kinds are explained by the evil workings of demons or wicked spirits who come into the sufferer's body. It is a short step from this to the belief that someone else has the power to drive that demon *into* a body. In many parts of Africa today, the problem for the witch-doctor is not to diagnose the *nature* of the illness, but the *cause* of it. He is not interested in the bruise on the stubbed toe, but who put the stone in the path of the injured foot. Contrary to popular assumption, not all witch-doctors are evil-doers. On the contrary they specialize in 'lifting off' the effects of curses, or in driving out bad spirits. The witch-doctor counteracts the effects of witchcraft, and may know a great deal about herbal remedies, diagnosis of physical symptoms, and understanding of mental disorders, which help him to convince the patient that he is truly able to cast out devils from a sick body to effect a cure.

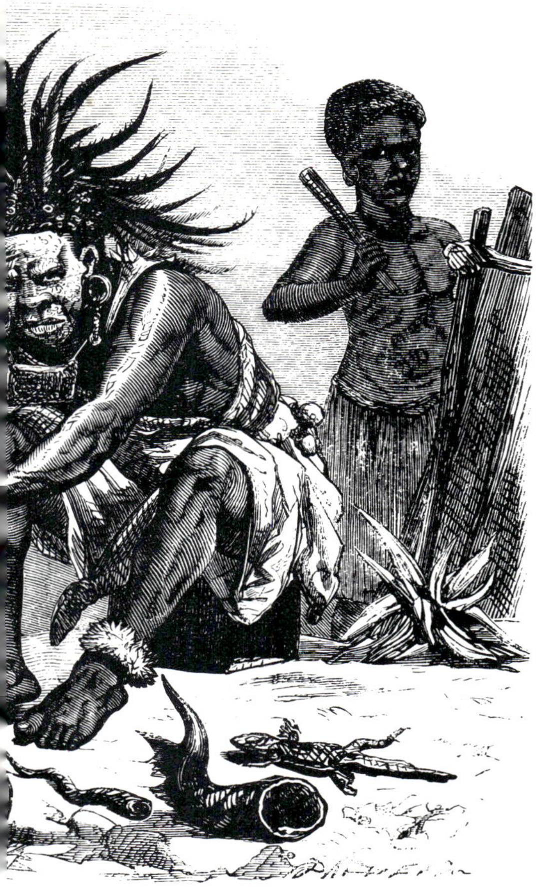

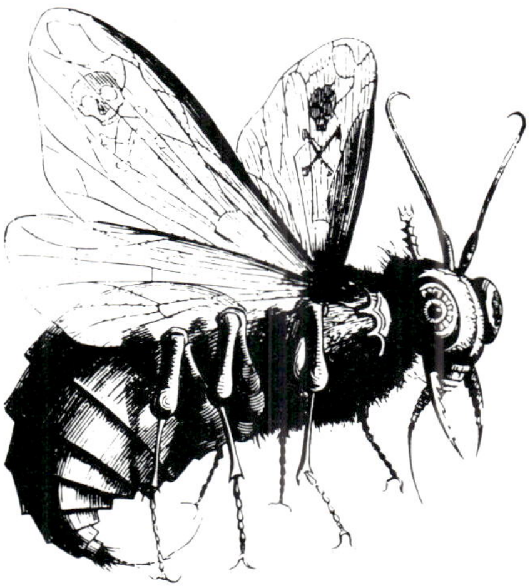

Left *Another demon, the fearsome Beelzebub, who took the form of a fly. The greatest deities were, of course, the sun and the moon.*
Below right *Idols of the sun and moon made from animal skins are worshipped by the North American Mandan Indians.*

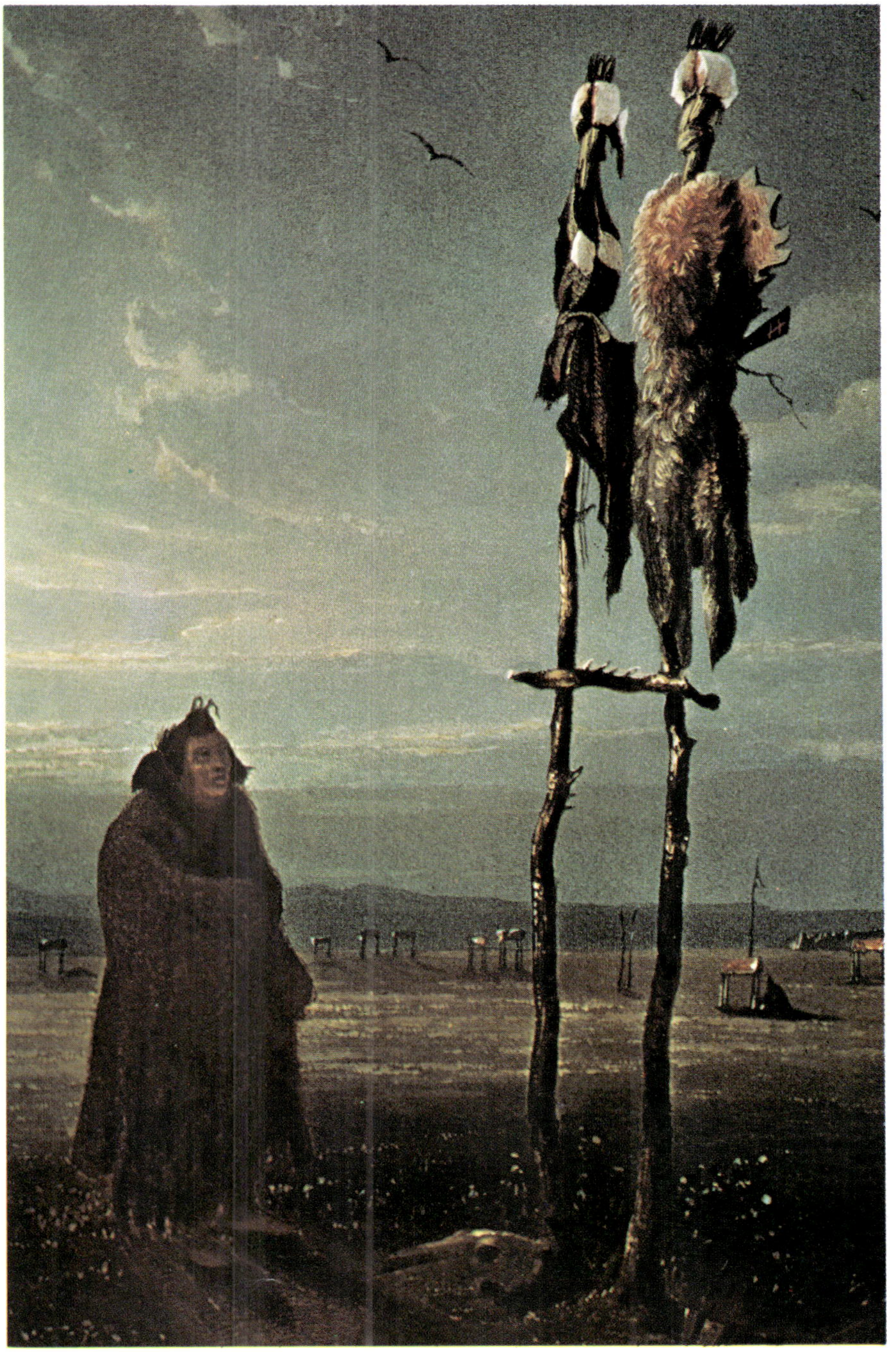

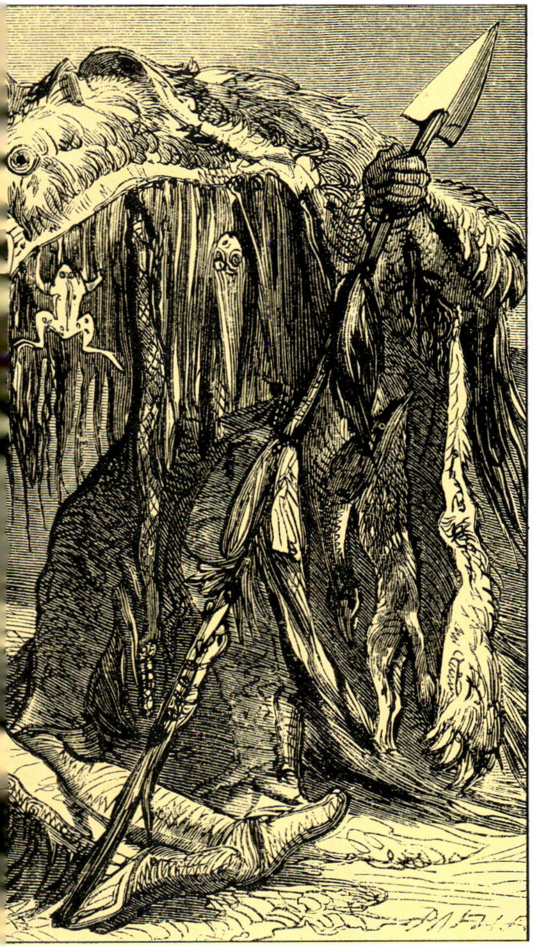

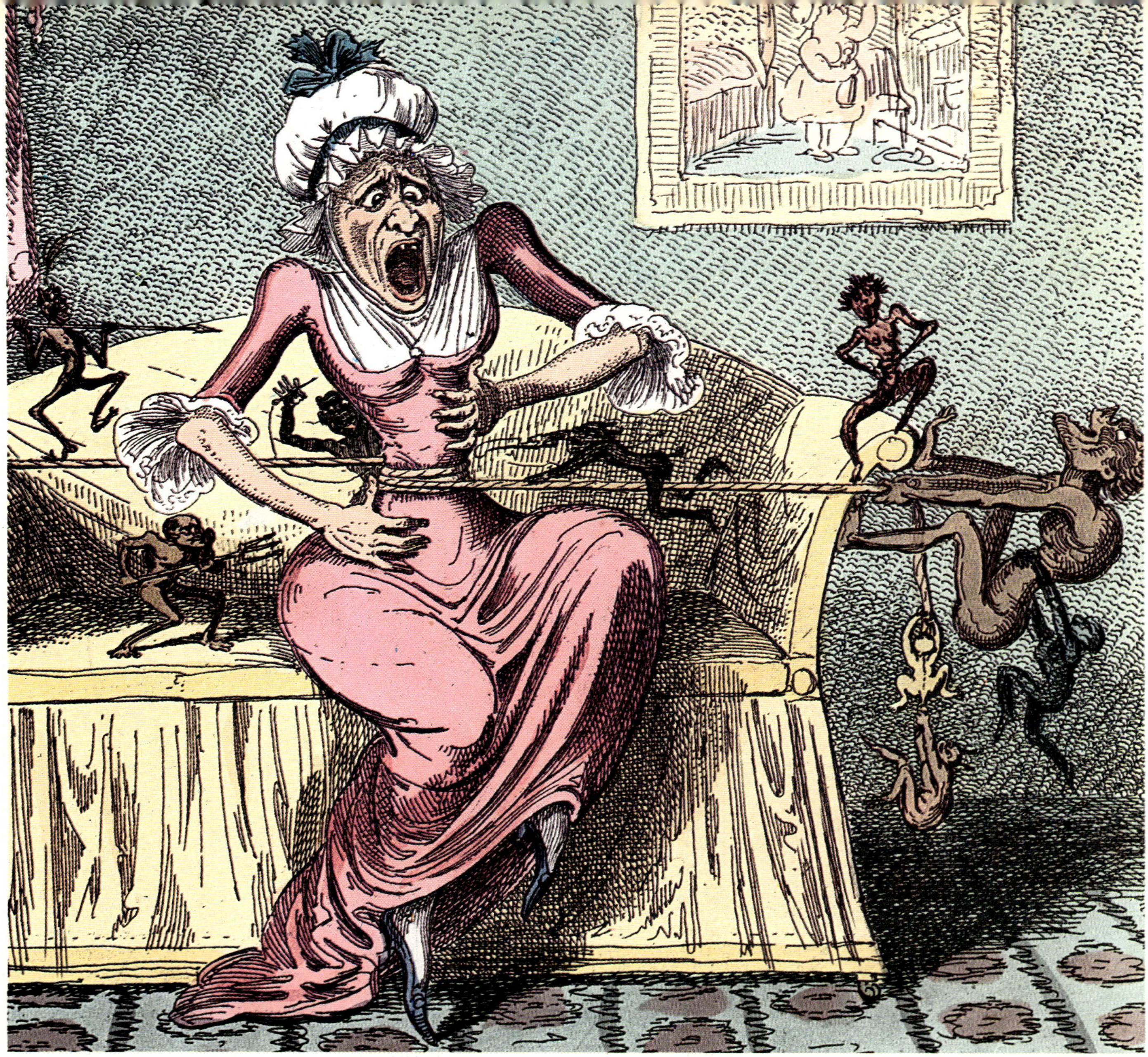

The theory that demons cause illness is brilliantly satirized in these nineteenth-century cartoons. **Above** *The pain of acute indigestion is inflicted by a horde of imps and demons pulling a cord tightly around the victim, while* **Right** *Another battalion of suitably armed imps cause a violent headache.*

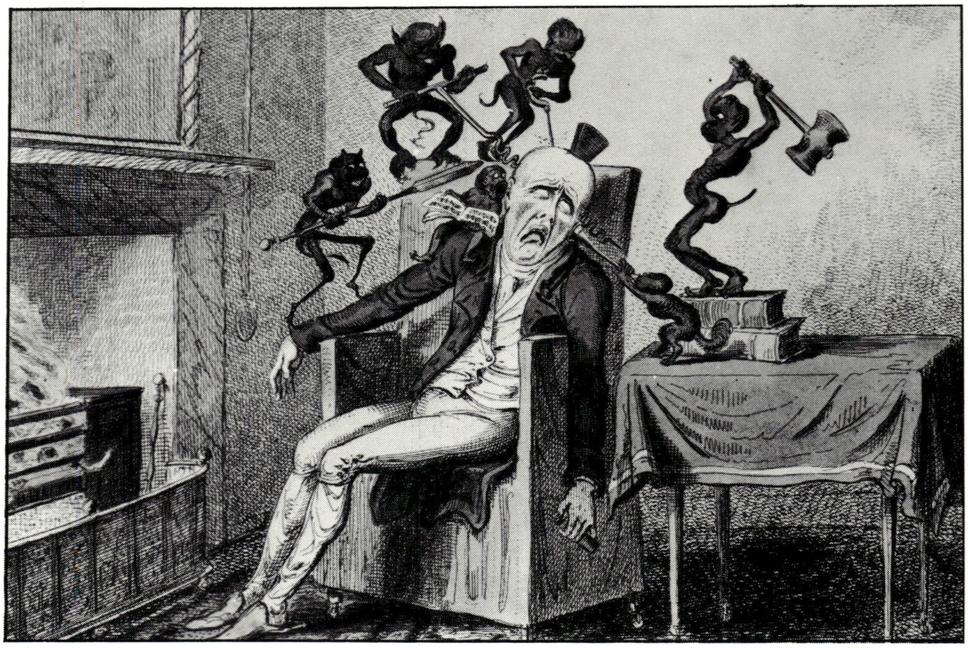

Medicine and magic thought

Medieval Christianity and demons

This association of the forces of good and evil with illness and disease is common to all societies, and lasts for a long time, even into what we would consider to be the civilized world. Demonology was a very important field of study for the priests of the early and medieval church. Scourging to drive out wicked spirits, in cases of epilepsy or for many forms of mental illness, was commonly practised in Europe until well into the last century. For hundreds of years, the kings and queens of England, who were appointed by divine right to their thrones, were supposed to have the power of healing, and often allotted special days in the year when the lame and crippled could come to receive the 'king's touch' in the hope of effecting a cure. Many traditional names for diseases show the age-old link with Christian views of illness as a curse from God: St Anthony's Fire and St Vitus' Dance are typical examples.

Gradually, explanations for disease become more sophisticated and complex. Just as it is possible for one human being to have the power to drive a demon into another's body, so also there are many special people who have the innate ability to effect cures. Over the centuries, almost any characteristic that is a little out of the ordinary has provided enough power to make that individual one who can 'work the cure'. Seventh sons of seventh sons; husbands and wives with the same surnames before marriage; babies born with a 'caul' (membrane) over their heads; strangers met at crossroads strangers riding by on white horses – all these and many more all over the world are attributed with healing powers.

English kings and queens were reputed to have the power of healing. Special audiences were given for the sick to receive the 'king's touch'. **Below left** *King Charles II is shown touching a sick man* **Below right** *These gold coins were hung around the neck to prevent sickness. They were called 'angels' because of the engravings on their heads. Gold is traditionally a healing metal.*

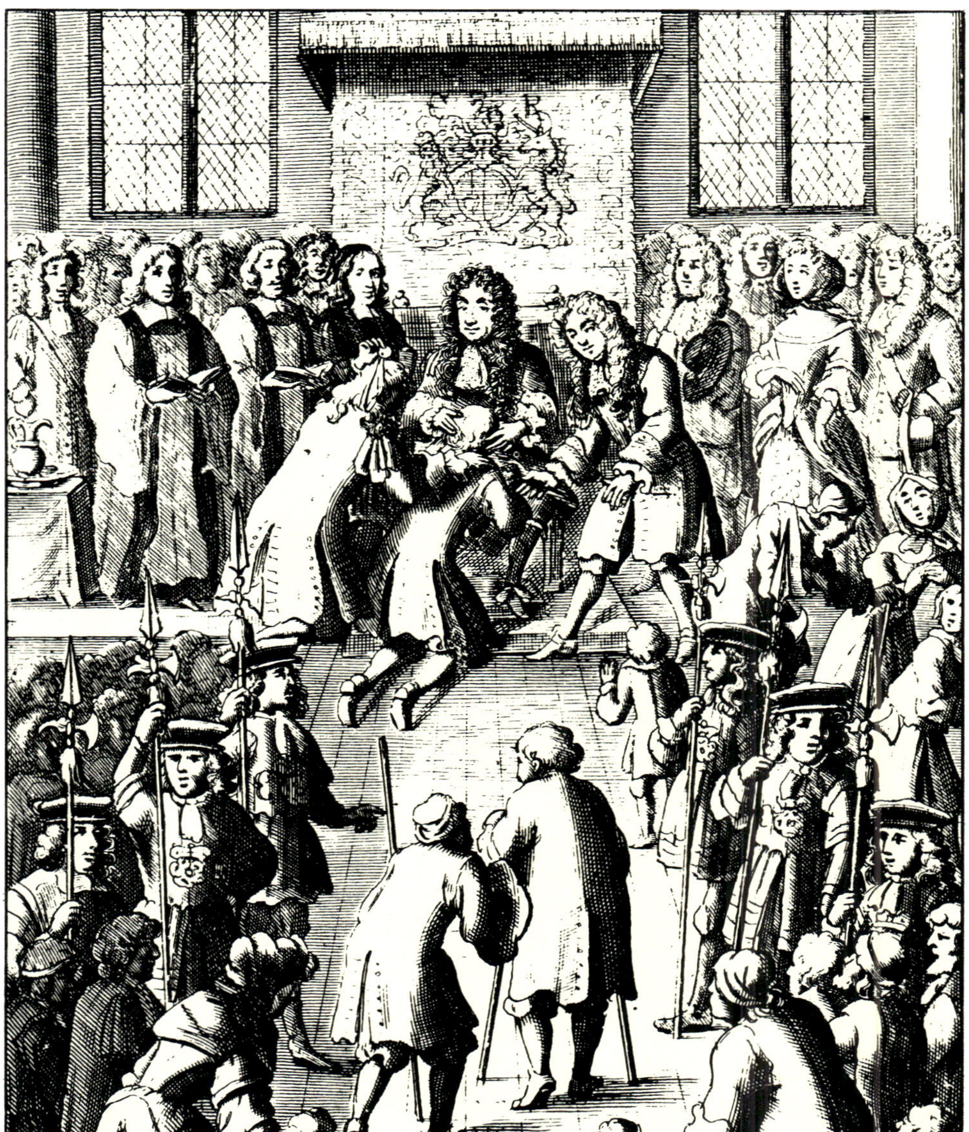

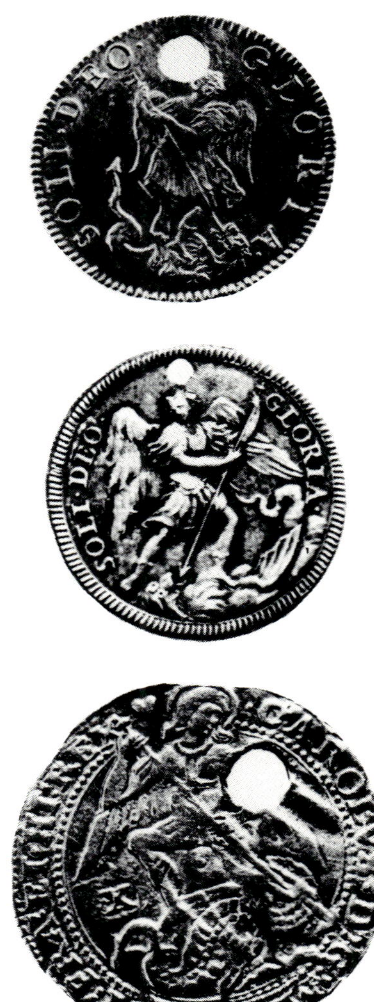

The power of dead matter

Even dead humans can work cures: powdered skull was considered a good remedy for epilepsy until the turn of this century in Scotland and Wales. A handful of earth off a dead man's grave would cure fits – provided it was collected at midnight. The touch of a dead man as a cure for warts, impetigo, running sores, etc is acknowledged in many parts of the world. It is interesting to note how many shrines or curing wells are established near the site where a famous person died or was murdered – saints particularly. As far away as China, bread soaked in the blood of an executed criminal is a traditional treatment for tuberculosis, while in Afghanistan walking round a grave and beating limbs with a reed branch is known to ease rheumatism.

Keeping the body whole

The 'wholeness' of a person's body is traditionally regarded as having a special power in itself. Care is always taken to prevent bits and pieces of it from falling into the wrong hands, Mothers still bite away long nails from their babies' fingers, and burying or burning cut hair is a living custom in many parts of the world – echoing the Old Testament story of Samson and Delilah. In many countries, 'wasting-away' illnesses are explained by the belief that some evil person has acquired a valuable commodity such as a lock of hair or a handful of nail parings, and used them in a curse. As long as the bits remain separated from the original owner, he is in danger.

Spittle as defense

A variation on this theme is that a man's spittle is a very useful defense against evil of all sorts – 'fasting spittle' is considered especially efficacious. Fasting spittle is spit from the mouth of someone who has abstained from eating for a specified period of time, or failing that, spit used first thing in the morning. Spit is universally acknowledged as a defense against the 'Evil Eye' – the curse put on by a spell-maker or witch.

In the Bible, Christ made a clay with earth and spittle to cure a blind man. In many African tribes, the medicine-man sucks at the patient's body in special places to draw out the disease, then spits it out of his mouth with a lump of spittle. Spitting on the ground after uttering a curse-word finds a modern lingering-on in the habit of spitting to indicate defiance or insolence, with no words spoken.

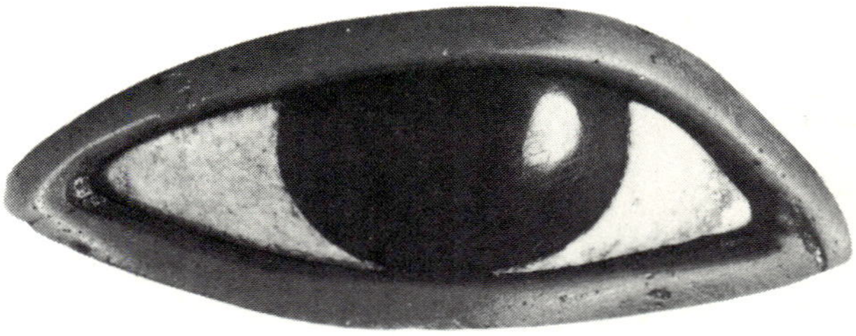

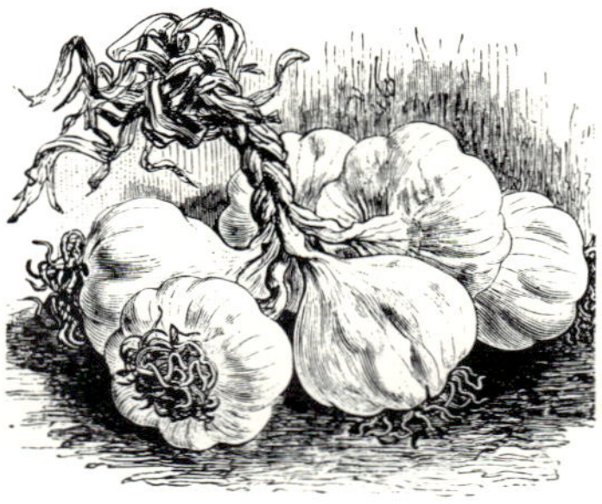

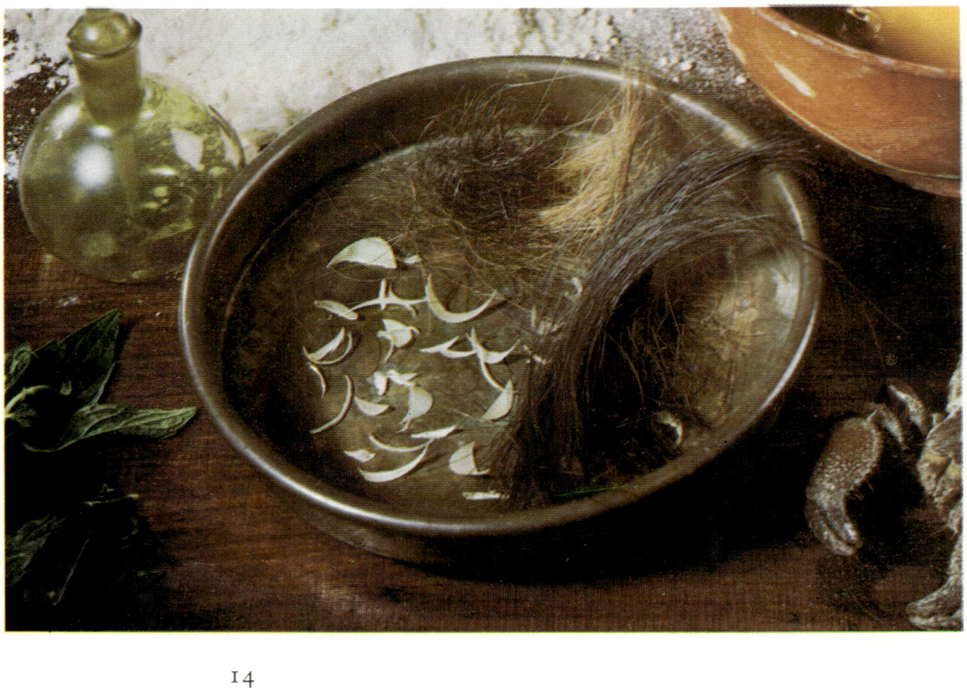

Above left *The 'Evil Eye' has long been feared as a cause of illness, inflicted through spells and curses.* **Above right** *Many herbs have been attributed with the power to ward off the 'Evil Eye'. One of the most traditional herbs is garlic.* **Below** *Bits and pieces of the body such as nails and hair clippings could be used in spells to inflict harm on the person to whom they originally belonged. Accordingly, many rituals for disposing of them are found in all cultures.*

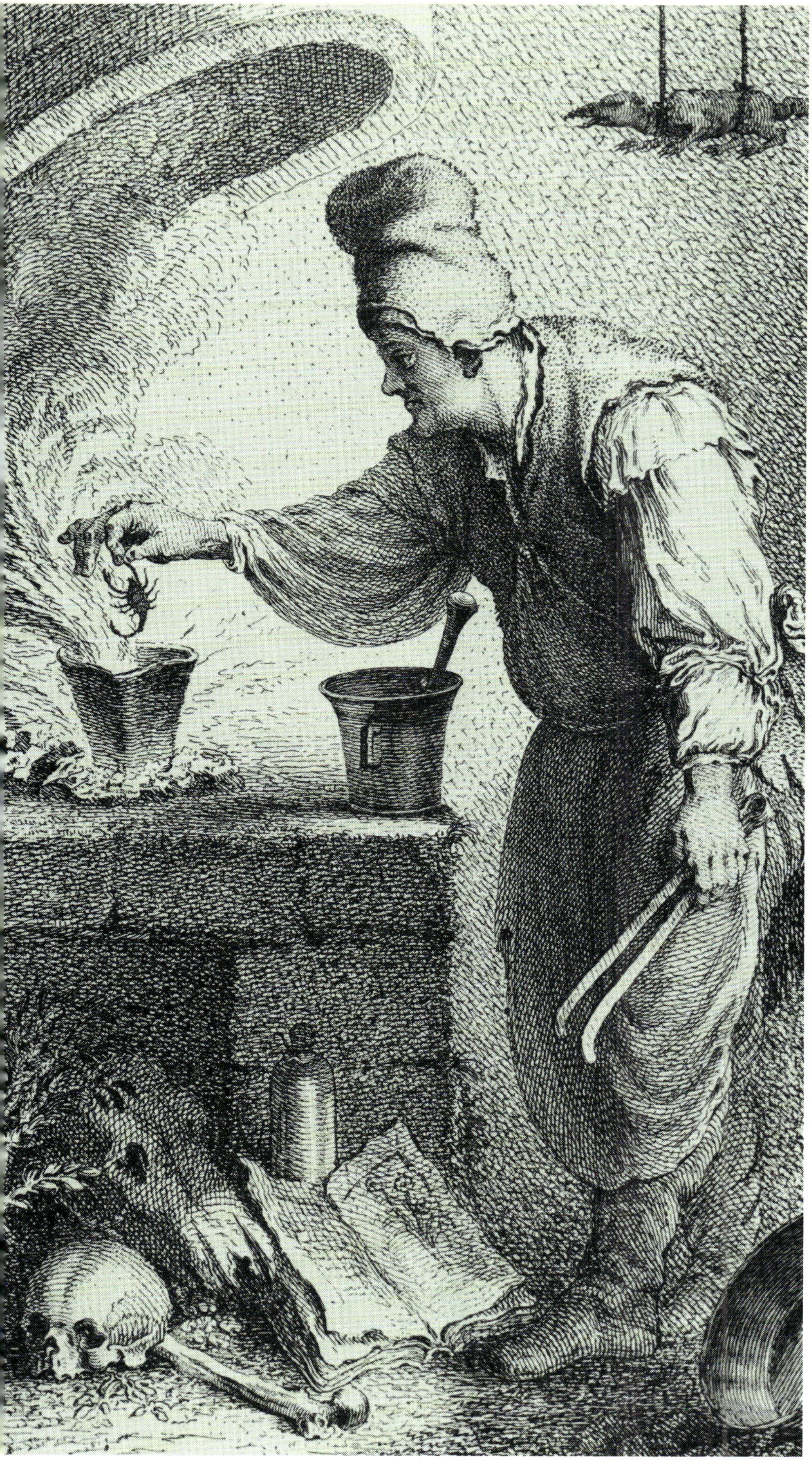

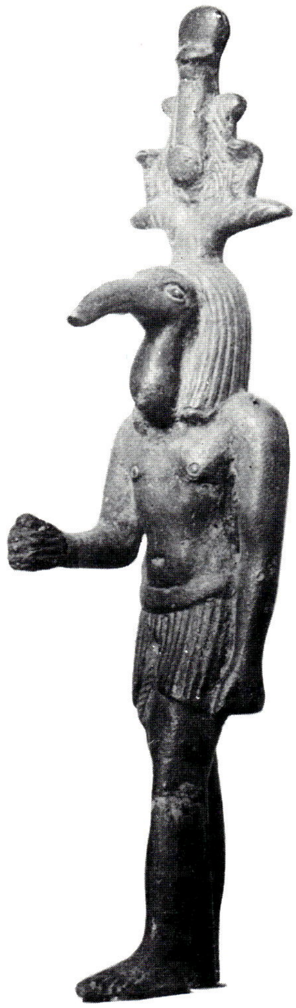

Below left *The most weird and wonderful remedies were evolved for potions to cure illness. They included such bizarre ingredients as powdered skull, scorpions, spiders and blood.* **Below right** *The ibis-headed god Thoth was the Egyptian deity who presided over medicine and surgery.*

Right *The dream of the alchemist was to create the 'Philosophers' Stone'. The Stone was perfect gold, which would cure all ills and make its owner immune to the power of death. The illustration shows one of the stages of its creation, in which the perfect solution is achieved by combining male and female elements in harmony.* **Below** *Coral, in the form of babies' teething rings, was believed to have both healing and protective powers.* **Bottom** *Plague was the scourge of man through the centuries, and 'cures' for it were constantly peddled to desperate people.*

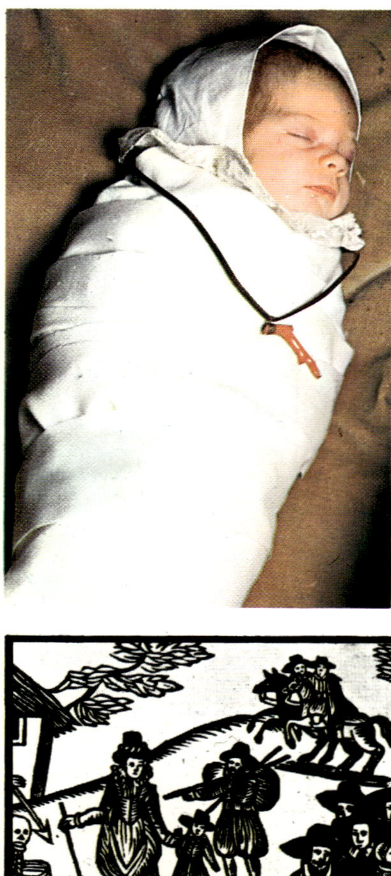

Animal and mineral cures

Sometimes, excrescences from extraordinary or mythical animals have been endowed with the power to work cures. The most famous of all was the bezoar stone, which was introduced into Europe by Arab apothecaries, and remained an orthodox remedy until well into the seventeenth century. It was a concretion found in goats' bowels, and supposedly provided an antidote to all known poisons. For centuries it held an enormous reputation as a protecting influence – an amulet almost – where there was any threat of fever, plague, pox or other pestilence. In time the same name was applied to other stones, such as the 'bezoar of Luna' (silver), 'of Sol' (gold) or 'of Saturn' (lead).

Other gemstones have often been imbued with magical healing powers. The most widespread in use is coral which is still traditionally used to make babies' teething rings, and was originally believed to ward off evil spirits from the cradle. Amber was protective against the plague, also adderstone, a piece of coralline limestone which when split open has marks like the coil of a serpent.

Perhaps the most intriguing of all stone-cures is the toadstone, supposedly gathered from the head of a toad and worn as an amulet. It gave warning of poison by changing colour, and was effective against snakebites. The biological explanation for the origin of this rare jewel is probably the presence of the pineal eye that lies at the top of the head of Saurian and Batrachian toads, under a cushion of skin. If such remedies now seem incredible and far-fetched, one only has to think of the claims made nowadays for copper bracelets, powdered gold, or stinging bees, to see that there is still a strong tradition in animal and mineral cures. Indeed, there is evidence to suggest that old cures are on their way back.

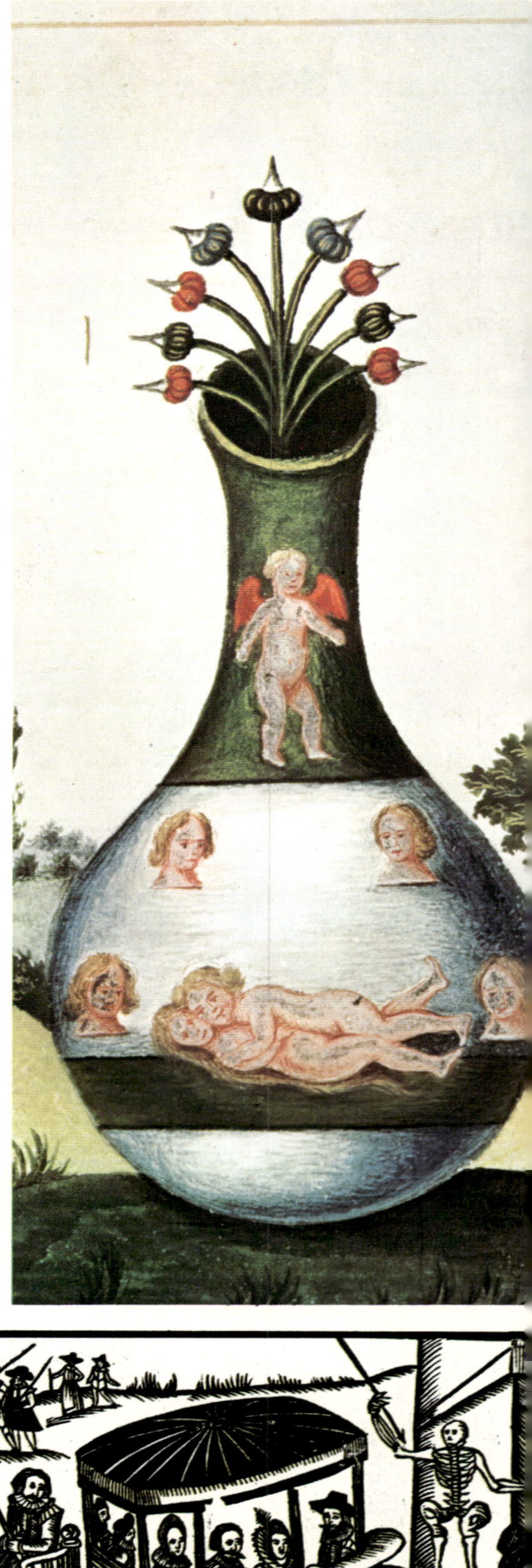

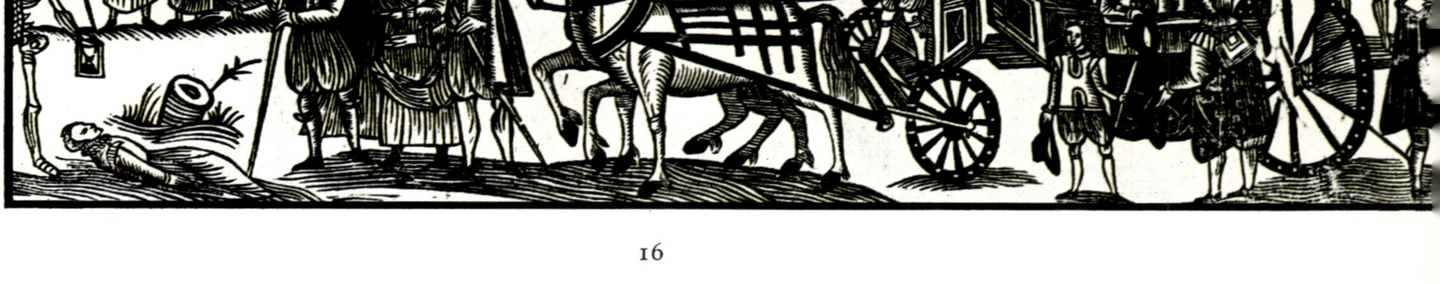

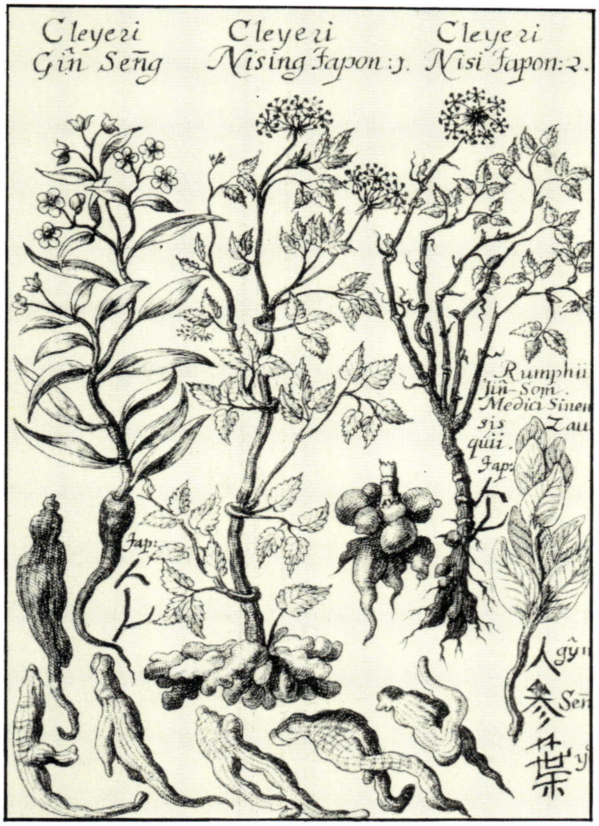

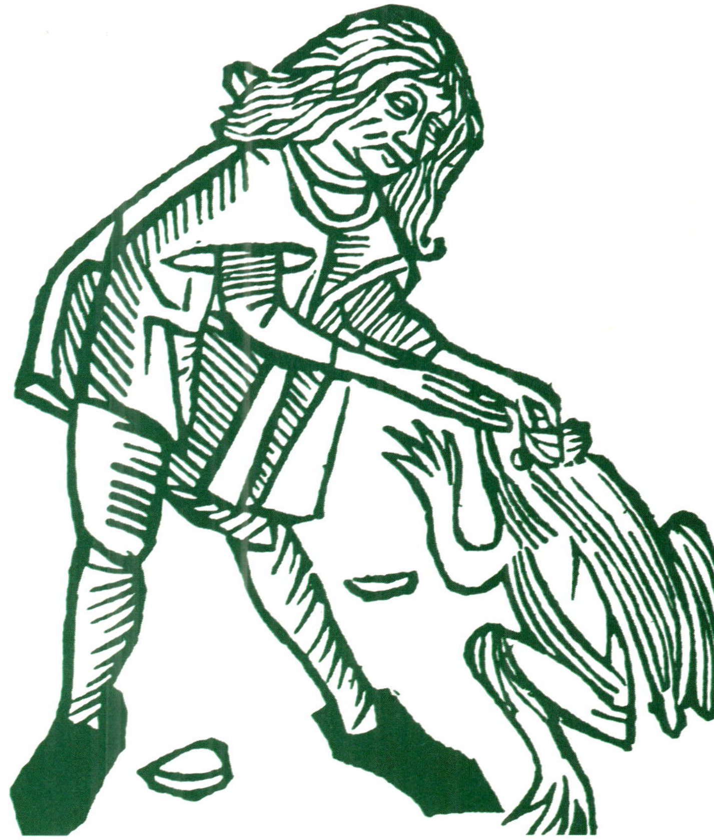

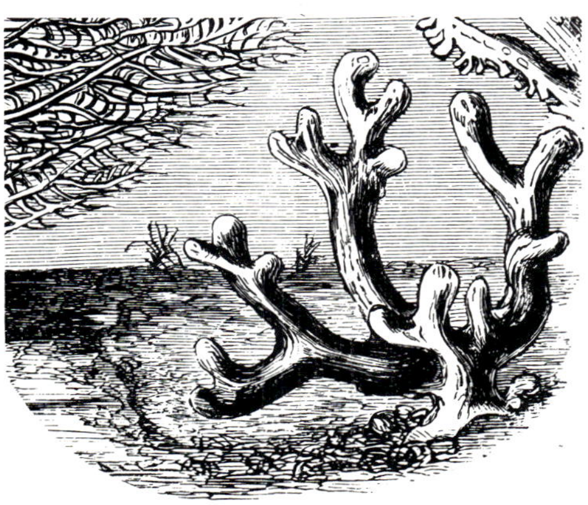

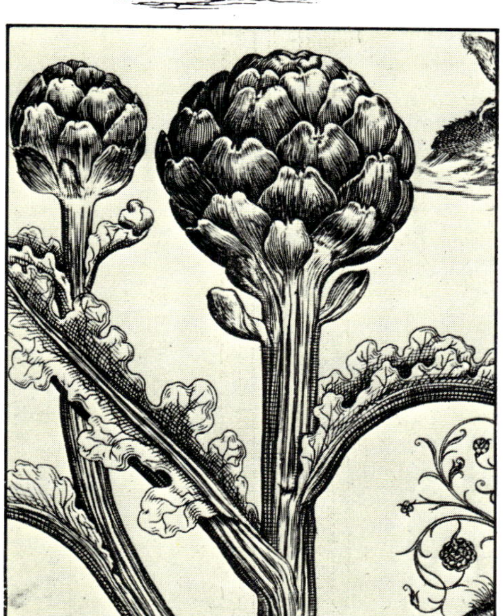

The doctrine of signatures

Many of the explanations for illnesses, and the supposed cures or curers just described rely almost entirely on the most important of all elements in successful treatment – faith. Every man with a desire to heal, whether witch-doctor or herbalist, psychiatrist or general practitioner, knows that the sick man will be healed most readily when he *knows* he will be cured.

Where no scientific explanation of a cause is available, then some other kind of explanation will be just as satisfactory, provided the patient is given a 'logical' reason for the cure. Perhaps the simplest and clearest demonstration of this is the 'Doctrine of Signatures', a system of natural healing that is found among widely differing societies, from the Indians of North America to the herbalists of Europe and the ancient Chinese. The basis of this system is 'like cures like': yellow plants cure liverish conditions, such as jaundice, which tinges the skin yellow; plants with heart-shaped leaves are good for the heart; plants with red flowers or blotches of red on their stems or leaves are good for the blood, and so on.

Many names for well-known herbs are

Above right *One of the most fascinating of all stone cures is the toadstone, which was thought to be plucked from the head of the toad, and was worn as an amulet.* **Above left** *The theory that 'like cures like' is reflected in the reputation of the ginseng plant, whose root resembles the shape of a man, and was regarded as a universal cure and elixir of life.* **Left** *Because of its colour, coral was reputed to cure blood ailments.* **Below left** *The shape of the artichoke may have accounted for its use in treating kidney complaints. This illustration is from a herbal printed in 1610.*

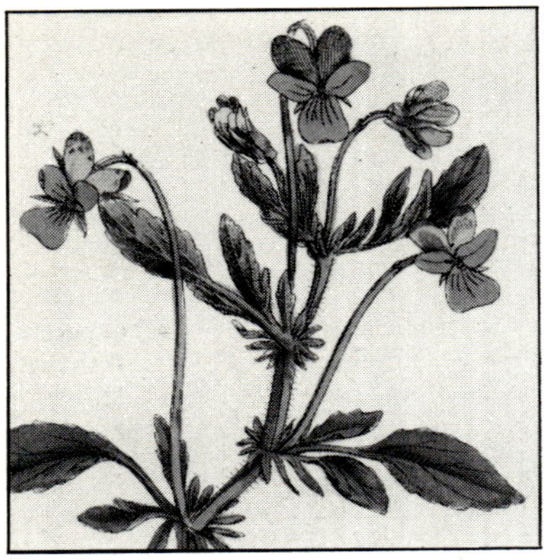

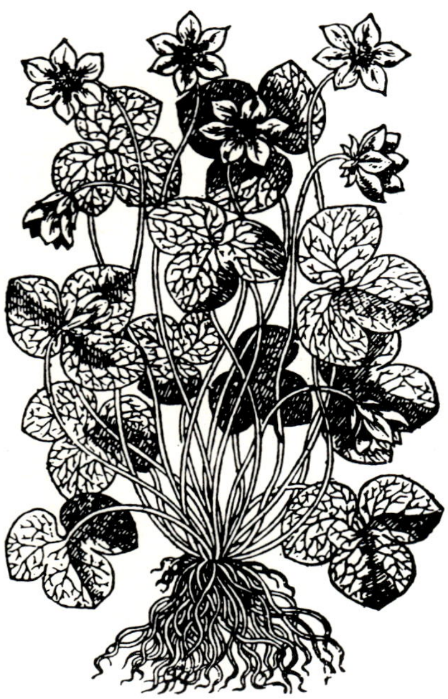

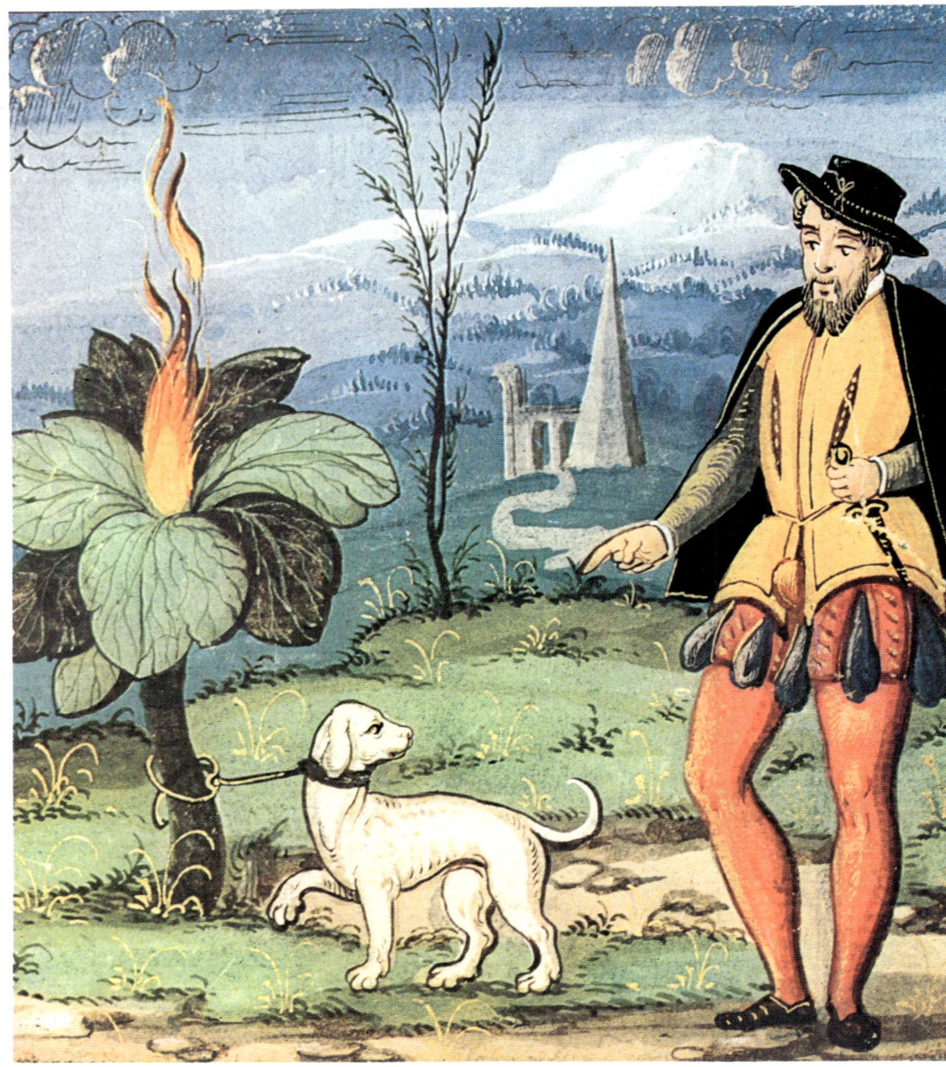

Above *The theory that 'like cures like' explains the common names for these medicinal plants, heart's ease and liverwort.* **Above right** *The mandrake, like the ginseng, has roots shaped like a man. A dog was traditionally used to pull it, because the screams of the plant were reputed to cause madness. It is also credited with universal healing powers.* **Opposite above** *Many people are really hypochondriacs, and try all sorts of remedies.* **Below** *One of the most important elements in healing is faith. Here, Jesus heals the eyes of a sick man.*

derived from this system of medical lore – heart's ease, liverwort, spleen wort, eyebright, are some examples. The language of signs extends to other objects besides plants: bloodstone has long been used as an amulet, for the red specks in the green surface are symbols of Christ's crucifixion, and the gem is supposed to stop bleeding if applied to a wound. The red colour of coral explains its use for blood conditions; emerald, in yellow green or white colouring, has always been associated with liver conditions; while the sun-like brightness of gold has made it a valuable cure-all for centuries.

A universal doctrine

To show how universally this system of connection occurs, there is the Hopi Indian cure of the weasel plant, used for women in childbirth. The root resembles a small burrowing animal, and as weasels pass through the earth quickly in their tunnels, a brew from the plant's juice was supposed to ease a baby's passage into the world. 'Seneca snakeroot' was also used by many different Indian tribes as a bite remedy, again because its roots resembled the snake.

At the other side of the globe, the Chinese used dried skins of spotted white snakes for leprosy, rheumatism and palsy; toads were used for boils, blisters and abcesses; and the famous ginseng root (shaped most uncannily like a figure of a man) has been regarded for centuries as a cure-all, an elixir of life. Modern scientists in China claim that this plant does in fact contain certain ingredients that make it valuable for the treatment of high blood pressure, diabetes, and general tonification of the central nervous system.

Faith in folk medicine

Fierce argument rages over the worth of folk remedies, and it must always be remembered that the magical or symbolic aspect of the plant or stone used in a cure was its prime virtue. Actual observation of improvement in someone's condition had little to do with whether a cure continued in popularity or not. To take one of the above-mentioned examples: the 'Seneca snakeroot' used by the Indians as a cure for bites was investigated by a young colonist-doctor, Dr John Tennent, in the early eighteenth century. He found the dried root was very useful for the treatment of coughs, and modern scientific analysis shows that 'senega root' does contain *senegin*, which is a cure for bronchitis, and is used in expectorant mixtures. What mattered to the Indian however, was his belief that the shape of the root was connected with *snake* cures. He could see it with his own eyes, and it gave him great comfort. This undoubtedly helped him to get better.

Where folk medicine succeeds

On the whole, folk medicine remedies survive longest when they deal with ailments which are of three types: 1 Short-term, possibly self-curing conditions, such as warts, some skin irritations, muscular aches and pains, etc; 2 Chronic or incurable conditions which have fluctuating periods of getting better or worse; and lastly, 3 Psychosomatic conditions, nervously induced states, such as coughs, headaches, rashes, or vomiting. In all of these types of illness, the state of the patient's mind is as important as the condition from which he suffers. Giving him something to believe in is almost more helpful than providing a physical cure. The condition will either heal itself, or come and go irrespective of the medicines used.

Where modern medicine fails

The survival of folk medicine or 'fringe medicine' alternatives to orthodox scientific methods shows in some measure the failure of modern medical systems to help people in the way most valued – with comfort and faith. One of our words for sickness, 'disease', after all describes exactly the problem of the moment: the patient is not happy with himself, and is suffering from an absence of 'ease' or mental tranquillity.

It has been estimated that 40% of a typical doctor's caseload at any one time is made up of conditions with a psychiatric basis. Any amount of chemical drugs will not cure these types of illness. While it is true that most survivals of folk medicine today are mostly in the nature of 'tried and tested' herbal remedies, it is only a short distance back in time before the symbolic or religious connotations of each cure come to light. No doctor worthy of his profession entirely dismisses the possibility of faith healing; the power of mind over matter is infinite.

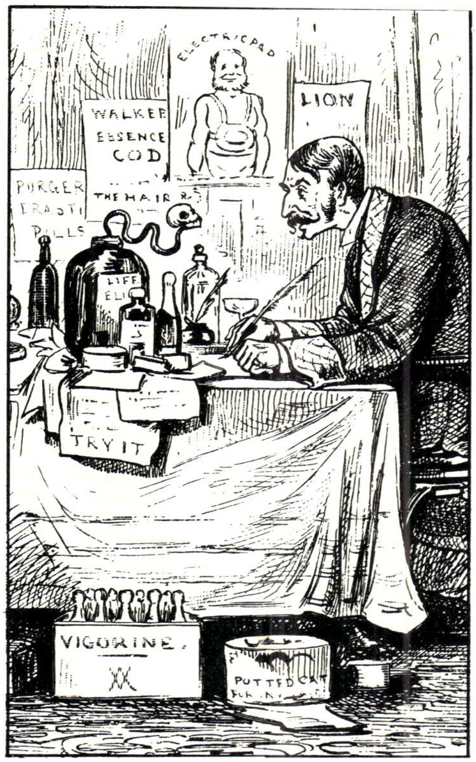

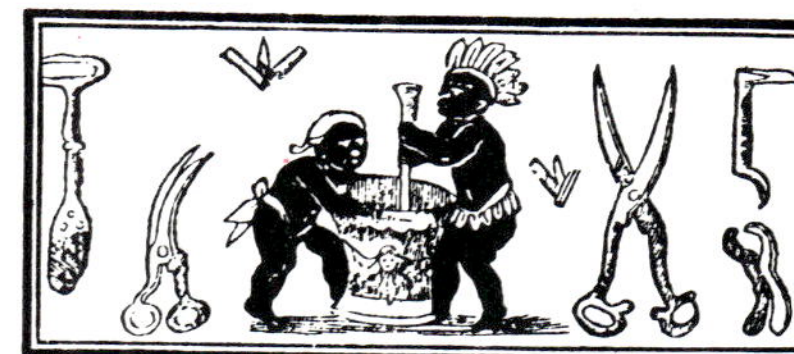

Good News to the Sick.

Veragainst *Ludgate* Church, within *Black-Fryers* Gate-way, at *Lillies-Head*, Liveth your old Friend Dr. *Case*, who faithfully Cures the Grand *P*–, with all its Symptoms, very Cheap, Private, and without the least Hindrance of Business. *Note*, He hath been a Physitian 33 Years, and gives Advice in any Distemper *gratis*.

All ye that are of *Venus* Race,
Apply your selves to Dr. *Case*;
Who, with a Box or two of PILLS,
Will soon remove your painfull ILLS.

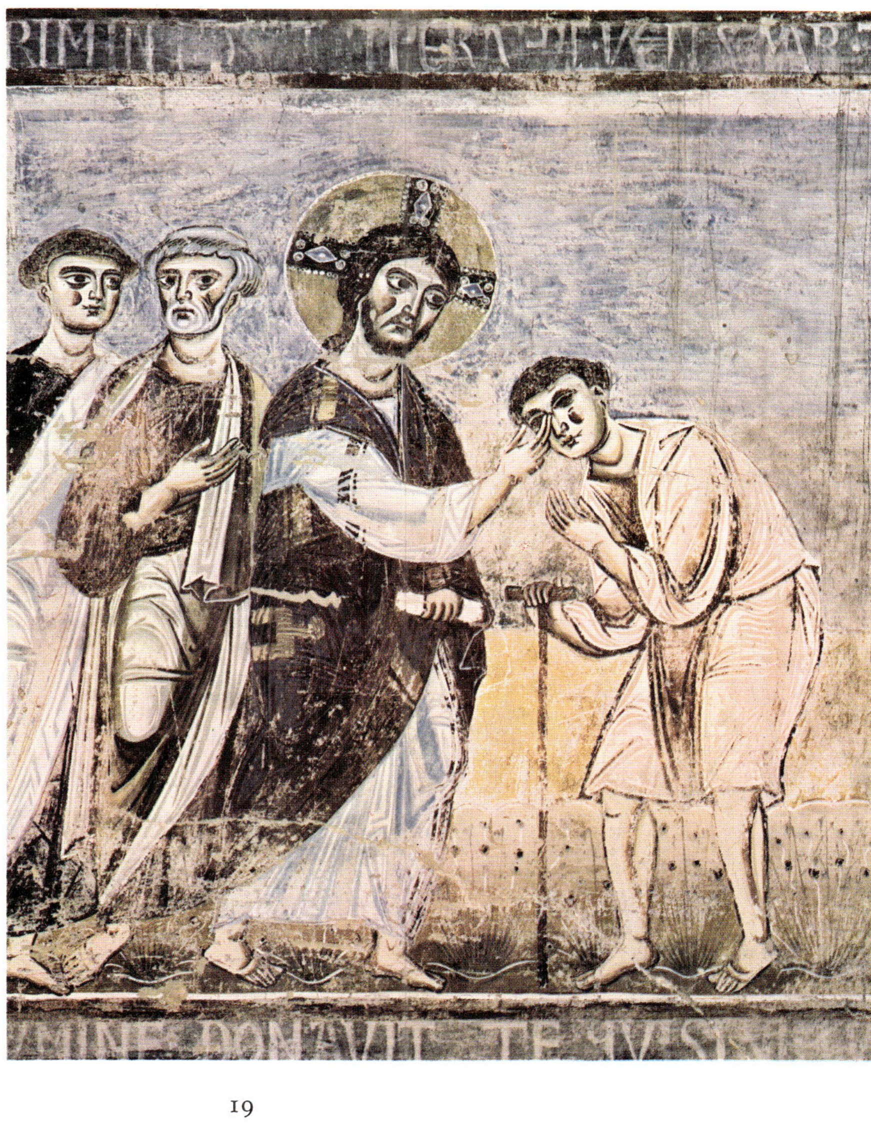

Above right *Myths about pregnancy often involve the idea of transference. For example, pregnant women traditionally avoided eating fruits with seeds in case they choked the baby.* **Below right** *A thirteenth-century manuscript of the female reproductive system also shows remedies for pregnant women.* **Below** *In the story of* The Sleeping Beauty *the thirteenth fairy brought ill-will. The illustration is by Arthur Rackham.*

Other theories of folk medicine

Almost as important in folk medicine as the 'Doctrine of Signatures' is the idea of *sympathy*. Once again, the effectiveness of this line of reasoning lies in its clear explanation. If a reaper in the fields was cut by his sickle, then he cleaned the blade, and hoped that the cure would be transferred to his wound. More familiar to modern readers will be the use of red flannel for rheumatism: the warmth of the colour was supposed to convey heat into the joint.

Sympathetic rituals in pregnancy

In many parts of Europe it is the custom to go round the house unlocking doors and opening windows when a woman goes into labour, as if the easy flow of fresh air suggests an easy birth to the baby. Malayan natives forbid pregnant women to do any net-making during pregnancy, in case the foetus gets tied up somehow. Canadian Indian women put aside all bracelets, anklets or necklaces for the same reason. In Scotland, women were traditionally 'unbraided' before going into labour. This survives to this day in the common warning to pregnant women not to put their hands above their heads (for example for pinning up their hair) as it causes the umbilical cord to wind round the baby's neck. We may have forgotten the 'Sympathetic' reasoning, but the actual prohibition is still widespread in all cultures.

Transferring cures

Linked to the idea of sympathetic cures is that of *transference* – which often involves some poor benighted animal! One of the best-known and amusing versions of this branch of folk medicine is a remedy for a child's cough, found in many counties of England and Wales. A hair from the child's head is mixed with the dog's dinner, in the evening. If

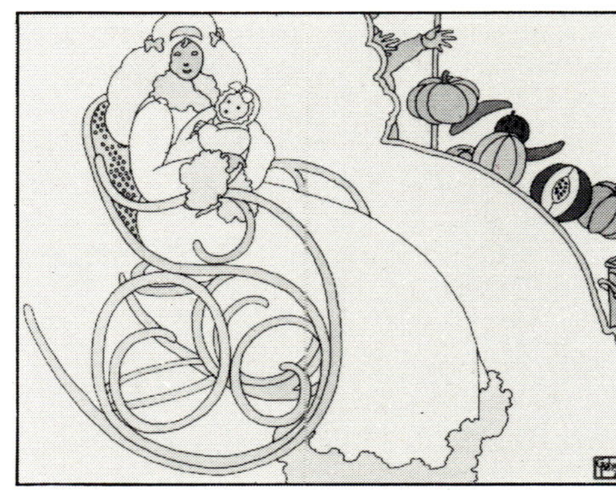

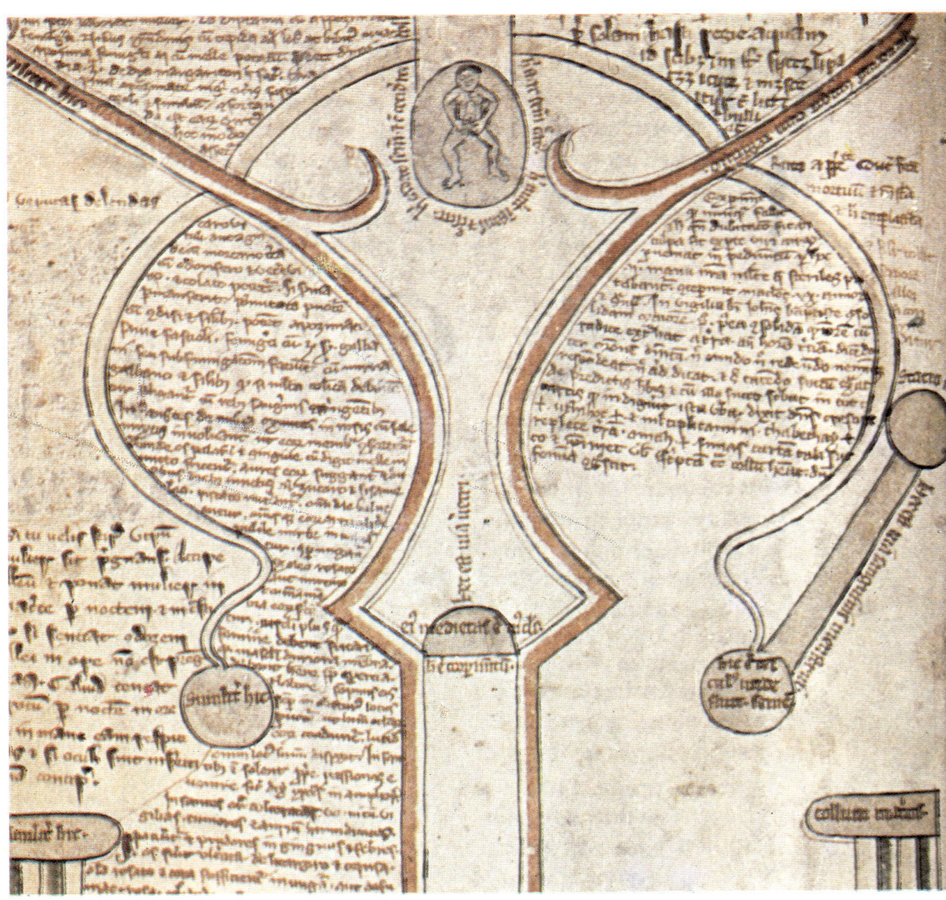

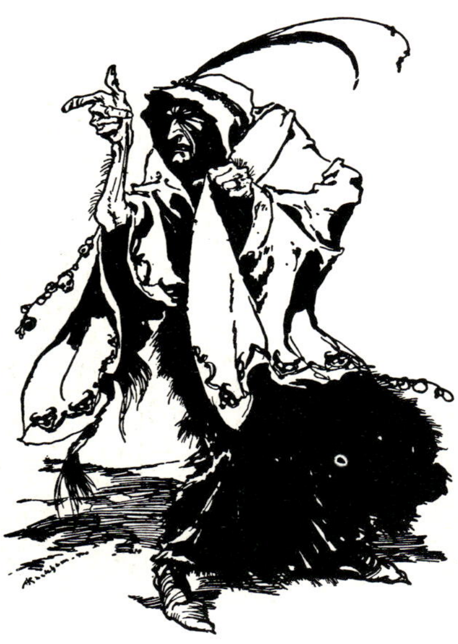

the dog chokes or hacks a cough while he eats his meal, then the child will wake up next morning cured! As many children develop a liking for a nervous cough, perhaps the sight of their pet taking it on convinces them that their own has 'vanished', and the compulsive tickle may genuinely be eased as a result.

Another dog cure is still with us in common speech: 'the hair of the dog that bit you' was for centuries literally applied to the wound. In different parts of the world hairs from particular parts of the body are selected, with the tail in general being more highly favoured. Further evidence of the 'Sympathy' theory survives in other expressions, like 'ears burning' when someone is talking about you, or 'itching palms' when someone is about to get money. In China, sneezing is traditionally regarded as a sign that someone is telling bad tales about the sneezer behind his back.

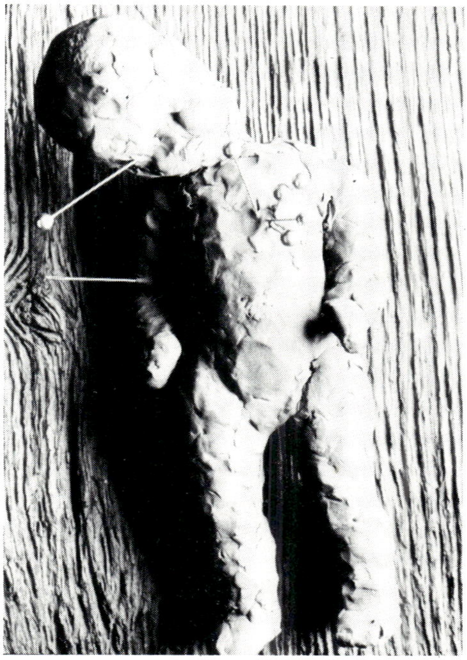

How transference can kill

The idea of transference can have a powerful effect on people still susceptible to its workings. Even today it is not uncommon for Mexican peasants to die of *el susto* or 'shock' at the sight of a doll pierced with pins or some other suggestive device. Western doctors can catalogue the stages of the illness, from the sufferer's description of '*se fue la tripa*' (my guts have gone) through actual stomach pains, diarrhea, vomiting, high fever, then anorexia (serious inability to eat) to languidity and indifference to normal life. Death can quite easily result.

One of the most dramatic variations of this pattern is found in the 'curse of the *veintiunilla*' or 'little 21', a popular name for a tiny yellow flower of central Mexico. If a victim sees this flower dropped into his dish of food, he knows he is doomed. He develops an insatiable desire for alcohol (entirely self-induced) and drinks himself to death, in the proverbial 21 days. Doctors will explain that he died of acute alcoholic poisoning, or pneumonia, which can so readily set in after a heavy drinking bout – but why the poor man is driven to self-destruction is only explicable by his belief in the power of sympathetic magic, and transference.

Transference and infection

An equally appalling manifestation of the transference theory has bedevilled attempts to check the spread of infectious disease in many parts of the developing world. In rural areas of India, for example, it has long been held that if a leprous woman wants to be cured, she should sleep with a healthy young man. One does not need to look so far afield either for other echoes of this same practice. Sexual assaults on young girls in order to cure venereal diseases were still being recorded in rural areas of England at the beginning of this century.

Another country remedy for tubercular or coughing children was to put them overnight to sleep in a cot in the centre of a sheepfold – so that the animals would take off the weakness. Holding live

Above left *Transference could be used to kill. The traditional method was to pierce a clay figure with pins or nails.* **Below** *Much of folk medicine abounds with the use of transference as a curing agent. For example, snails were traditionally believed to cure warts.*

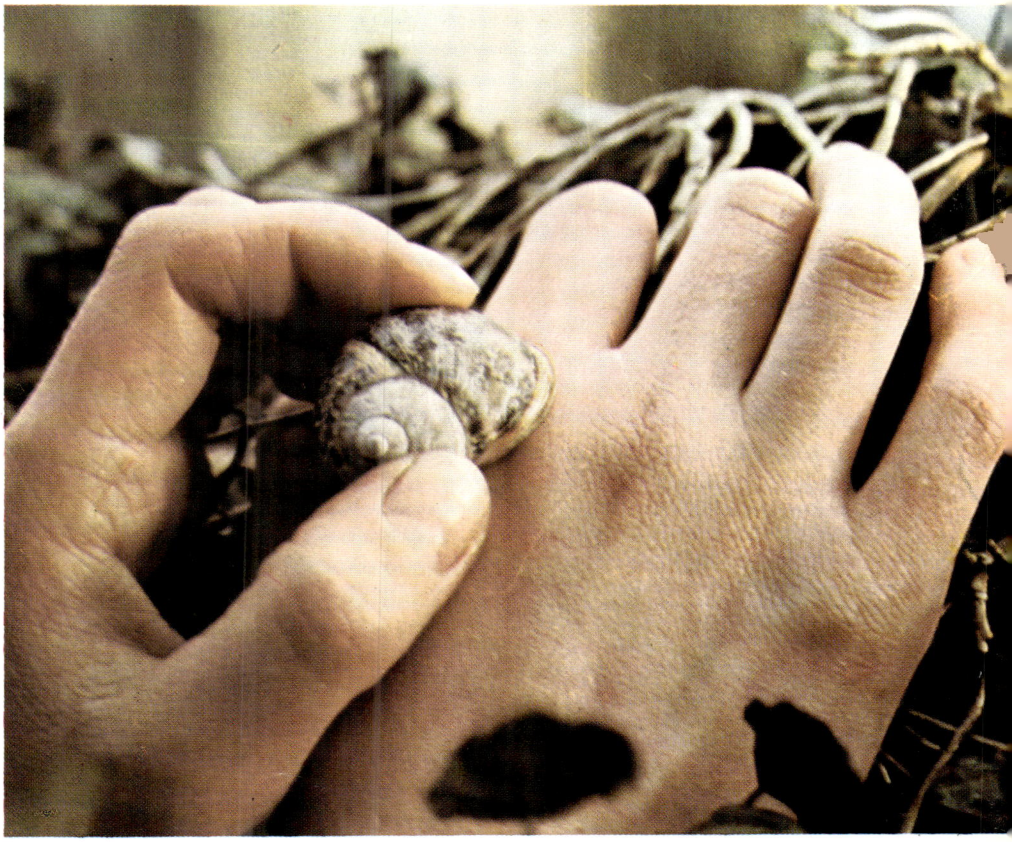

animals to infected parts of the body is supposed to have the same effect – frogs or toads popped into the mouth for sores and ulcers; spiders worn in little boxes around the neck for relief of the ague or rheumatism. Rubbing a cat's tail on a stye is supposed to cure it, and in olden days cats were supposed to kill babies by 'sucking their breath' – possibly explained by the association of cats with witches, and also by the sad and inexplicable occurence of cot-deaths in tiny children.

Other forms of transference

Transference of a disease need not necessarily be to an animal – it can be to an inanimate object or to a particular person. Many a schoolchild will remember the odd practice of 'telling' warts away, simply by whispering about them to another schoolfriend or an old aunt; a Cheshire wart remedy is to rub the lump with a bit of bacon fat then to slip it under the bark of an ash tree. In America, Ireland, and England, a cure for toothache is to drive a nail into an oak tree or into the beam of a cottage ceiling. Even the dead have their uses: boils can be cured if they are poulticed for three days and nights, and then the dressings are put in the coffin for burial.

Transference can work the other way round too: the phrase 'hare-lip' for a minor disfigurement in new-born babies echoes the folk belief that a pregnant woman is subject to 'impressions' during the nine months of carrying: either a hare ran across her path, or she put her foot unsuspectingly into a hare's lair. Hunters pull the scut or tail out of a hare before carrying it home, in case they come across a pregnant woman.

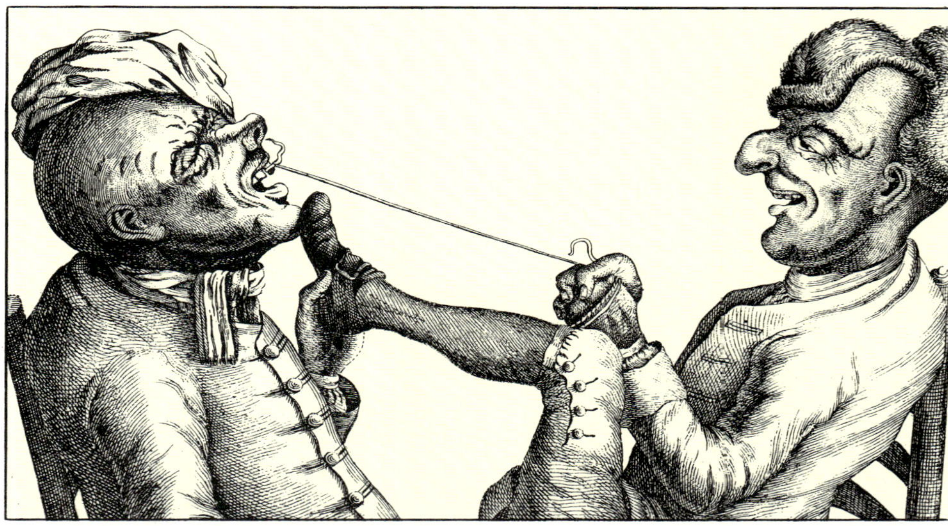

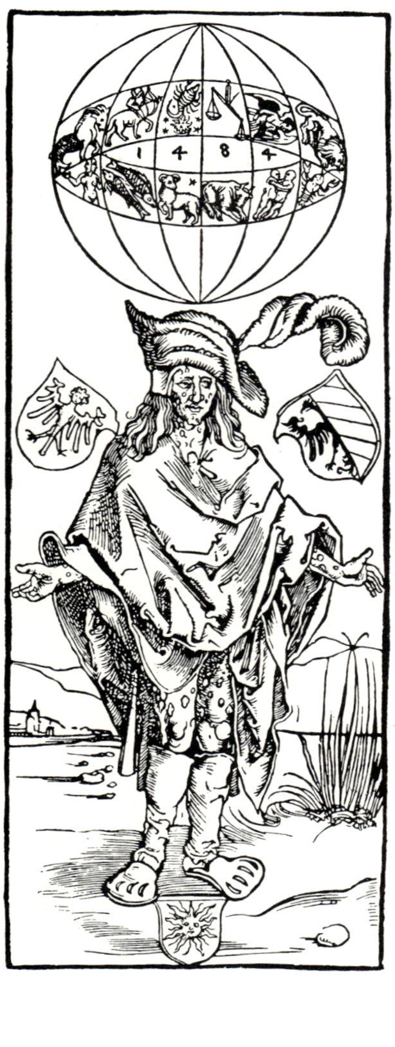

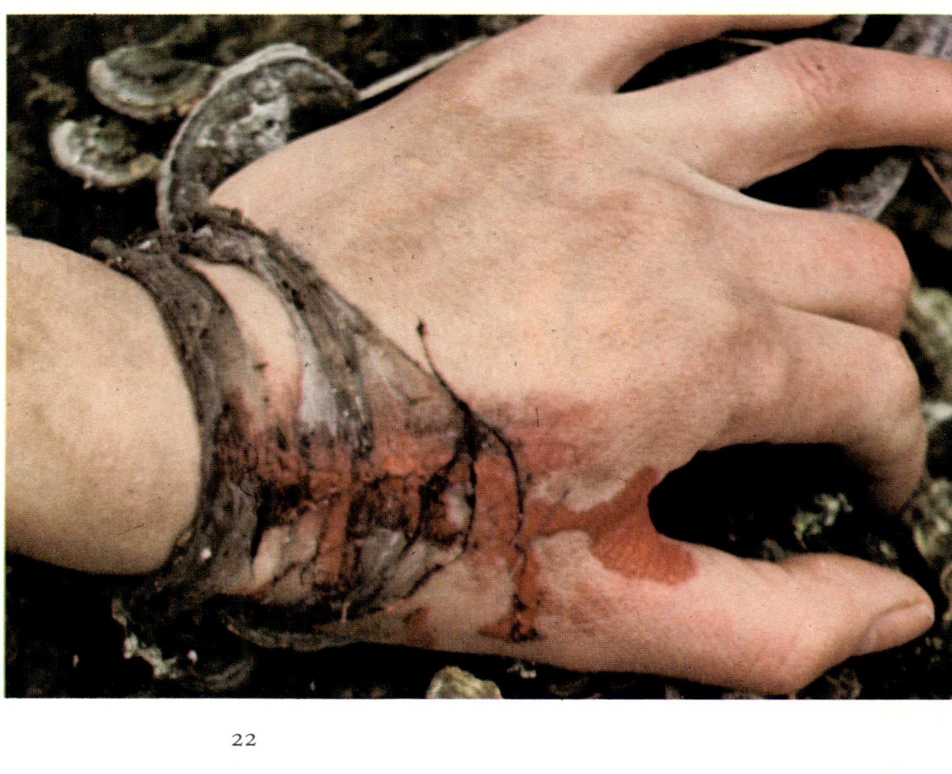

Above right *This is a painful method of curing toothache. A much gentler way is a traditional transference remedy, in which a nail is driven into an oak tree or a wooden beam.* **Below right** *A folk method to stop bleeding is to put cobwebs on a cut. The idea may have grown because the fine filaments of the spider's web look like the sticky fibrin threads that appear in newly clotted blood.* **Below** *Syphilis was thought to be cured by sleeping with an uninfected person to 'transfer' the disease. Of course this transference cure simply spread it further.* **Opposite above** *Midsummer festivals were held to appease the gods of nature. Gods and fairies were thought to appear to men. The illustration is for* A Midsummer Night's Dream. **Opposite below** *Over the years herbalists acquired a vast store of knowledge about the cultivation and uses of herbs.*

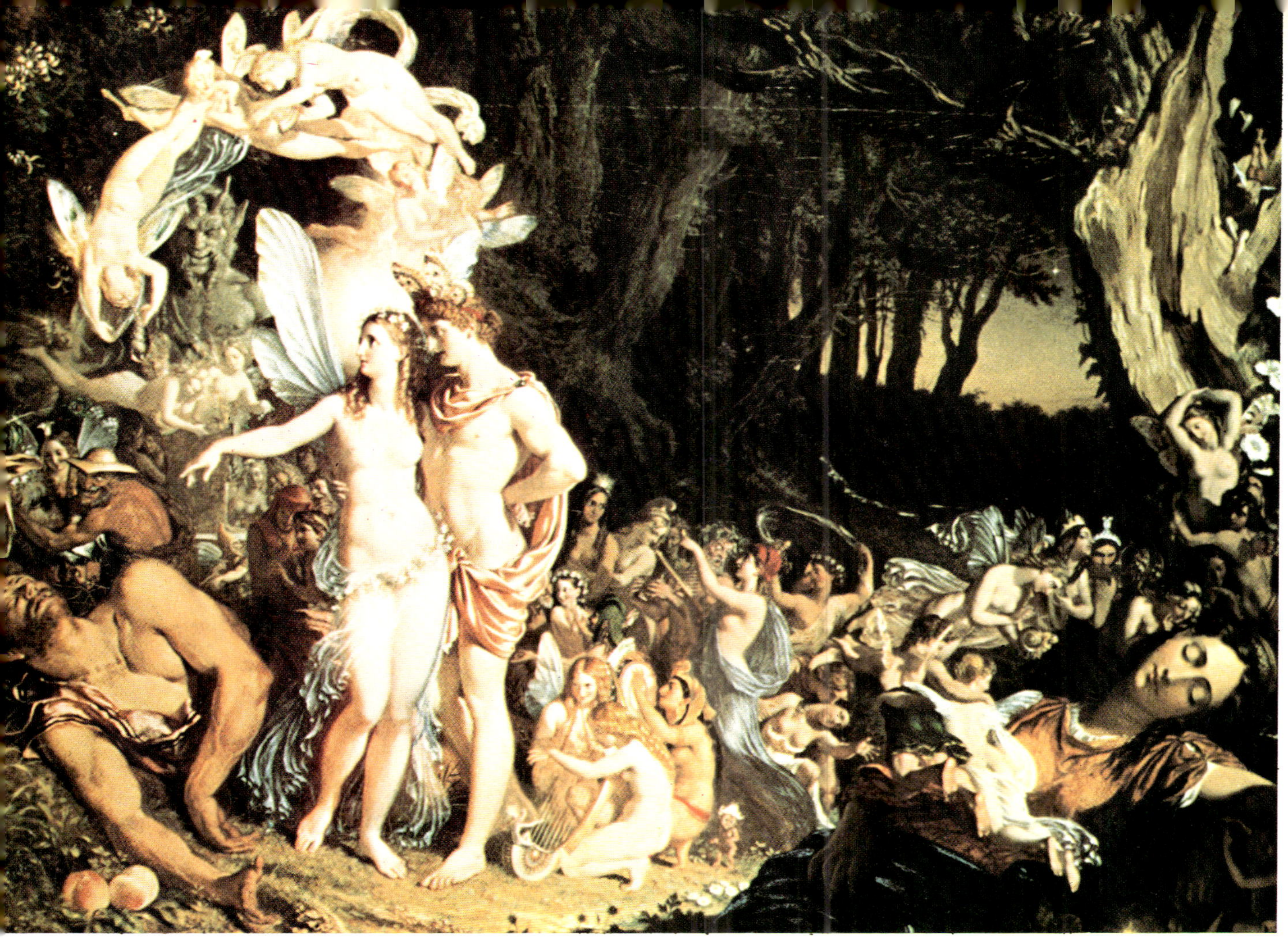

Outside influences on cures

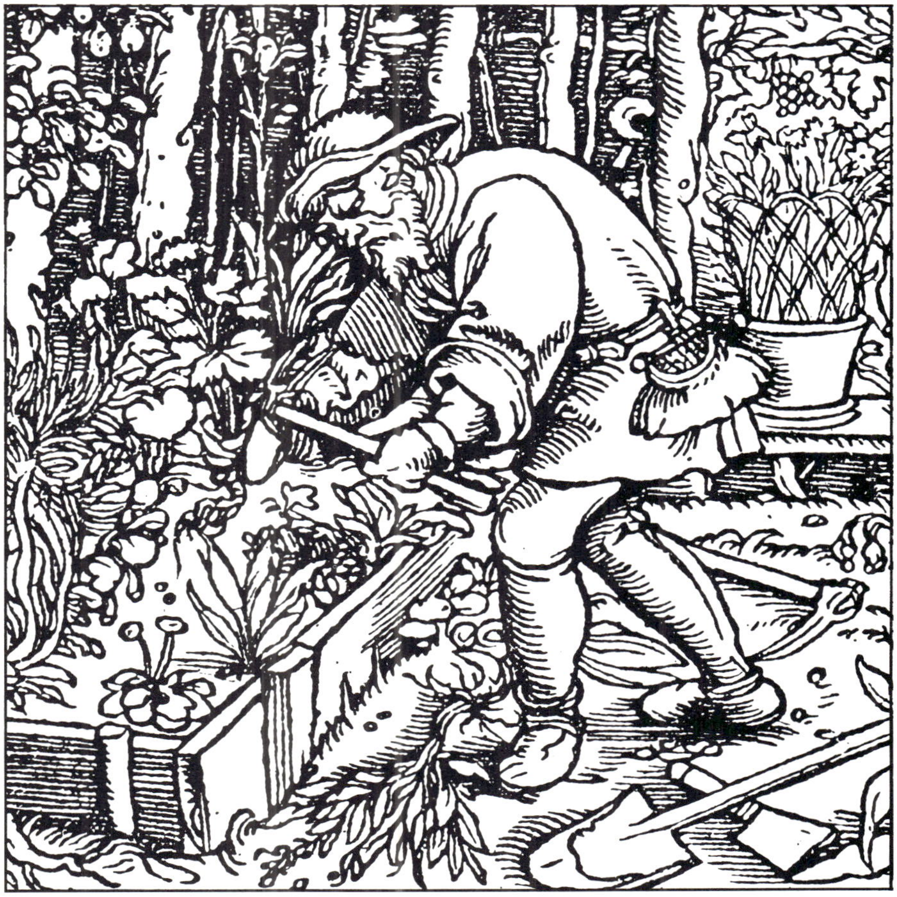

The logic which governs these folk cures and supposed associations between nature and disease is also applied to methods of treatment in folk medicine. Everything has its place in the order of the world, and there is an appointed connection between the ailment and the remedy, whether symbolic or sympathetic. There is actually a great deal of common sense in these rules or regulations about the gathering and preparation of medicines, for they demonstrate a real understanding of the way that things grow. Roots of annuals for instance, should be gathered in spring, before all their strength goes into flowering. Biennials or perennials are picked in late autumn, when storing their nutrients before winter.

Inevitably, many of the systems that apply to folk remedies are much more to do with magic, religion, or superstition of some kind, dating far back to the earliest periods of our history. Take the special importance of the oak and the mistletoe: in pagan times in England, midsummer

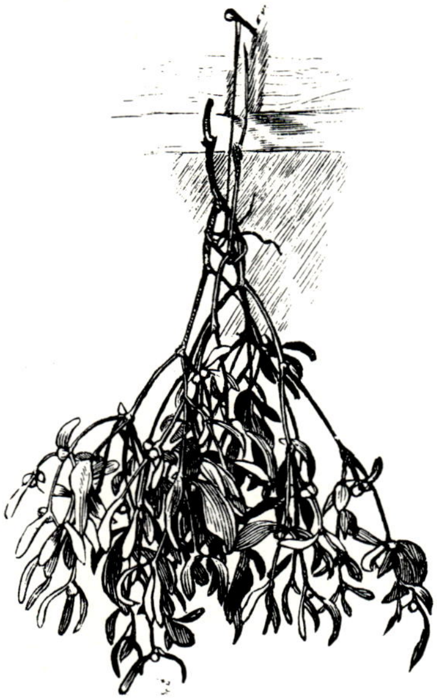

fires of these were made, often as an adjunct to an animal sacrifice at the height of the growing season to propitiate the nature gods.

The idea was to 'act out' a death in nature, so that the fields of crops around the village would not die. Mistletoe was particularly valued because it is evergreen and grows on seemingly wintry-dead branches. (French doctors in 1927 isolated a substance called *guipsine* from mistletoe, which for a while enjoyed a vogue as a reliever of arterial hypertension.) With the coming of Christianity, the fires continued but the purpose was shifted to something more respectable – the martyrdom of St John – for the saint's day occurs at this season. All the plants and herbs blooming at this time were now named for the saint – on 'St John's Eve' the spirits of the dead wander the earth again, and this is an especially good time for doctors to gather their plants 'alone and in fear and in silence' as the old herbals commend.

Planetary influences

In medieval herbal books, there are literally dozens of elaborate instructions covering the planetary influences at work on the natural world, and how certain herbs should only be gathered when particular astrological signs are in the ascendant. This school of herbalism found its greatest exponent in Nicholas Culpeper, who wrote his famous herbal in the seventeenth century. A typical instruction reads: 'If a man gather vervaine the first day of the New Moon, before sun rising, and drinke the juyce thereof, it will make him avoid Lust for seven years.' It seems fairly sensible that plants to be used for their juices are best gathered at night, with thick dew on them, whereas leaves needed for drying and crushing are picked on a sunny day.

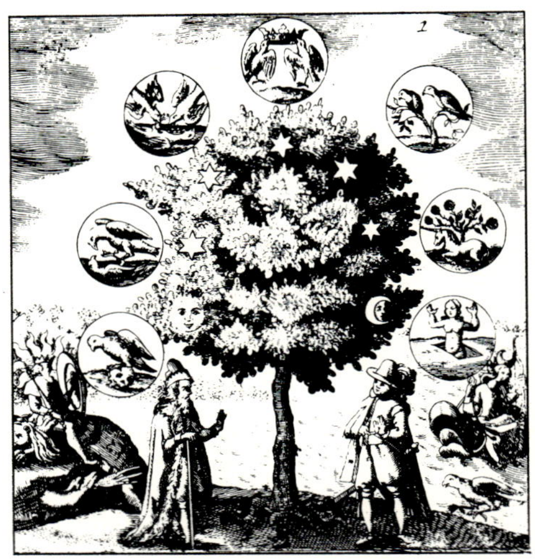

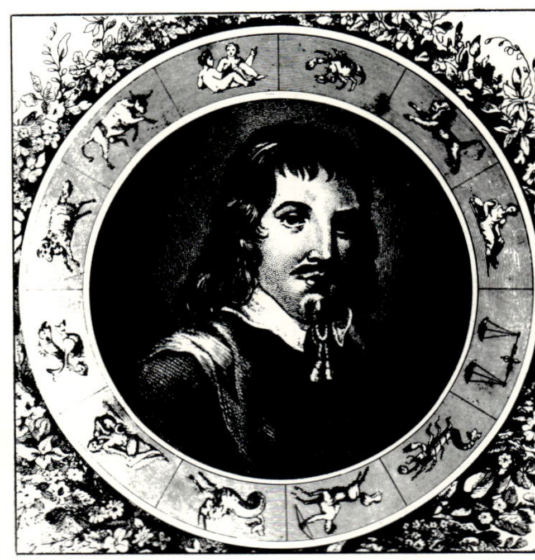

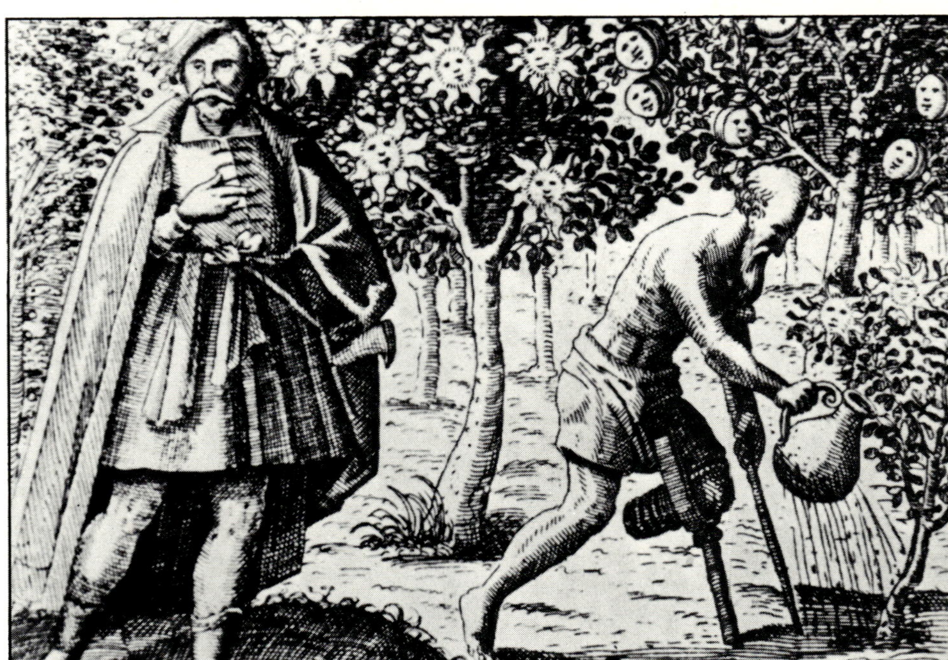

Above *Mistletoe was revered and used in midsummer fertility festivals because it lives on seemingly dead, wintry branches.* **Above right** *Nicholas Culpeper was the leading exponent of the theory that the planets influenced the natural world.* **Above left** *The alchemical tree also expresses the connection of earth, man and the planets.* **Below** *The trees in this garden bear the symbols of the sun and moon on their branches.* **Opposite page** *The zodiac follows the course of the planets, and they govern the activities of each season throughout the year.*

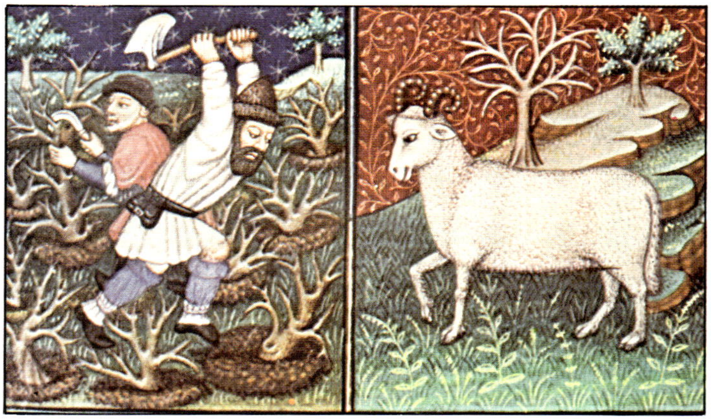

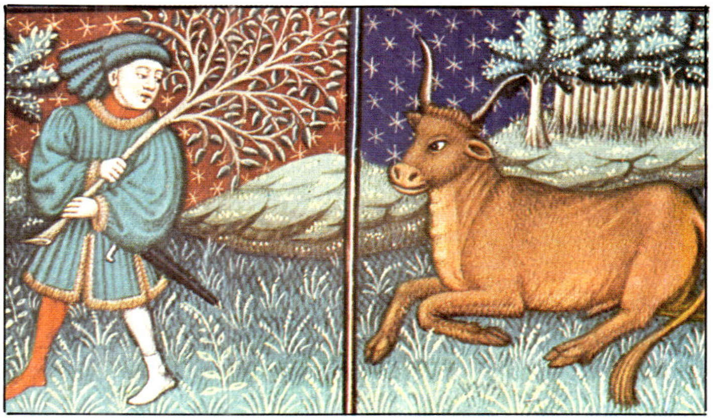

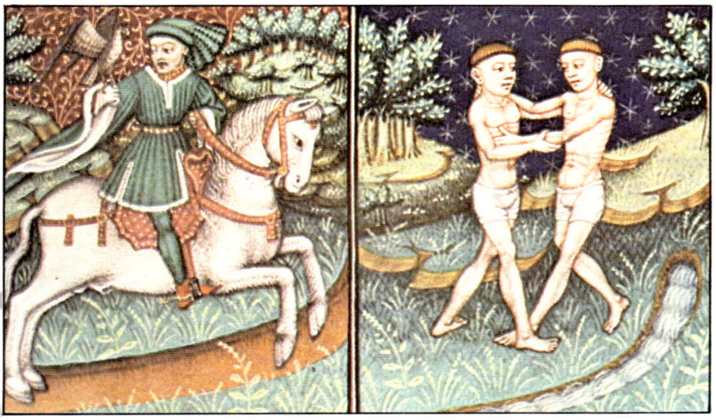

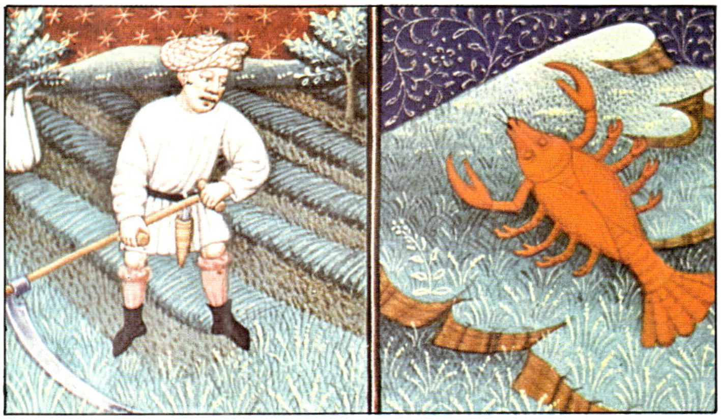

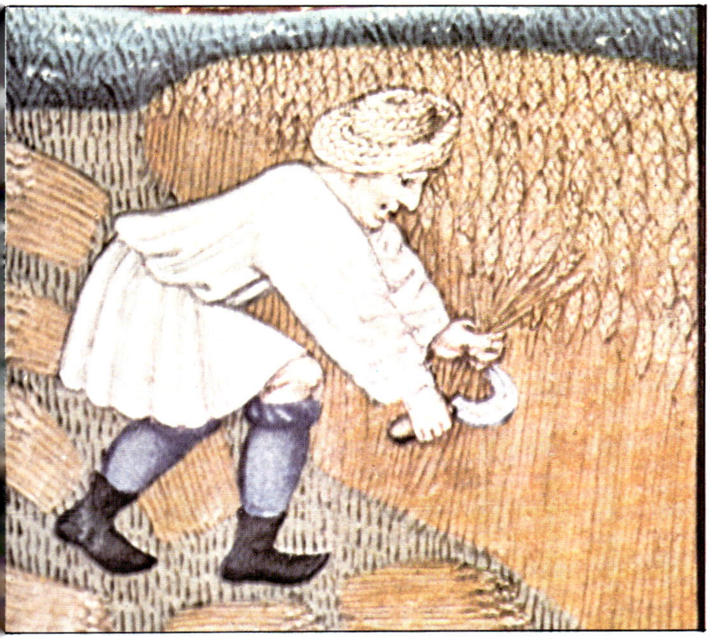

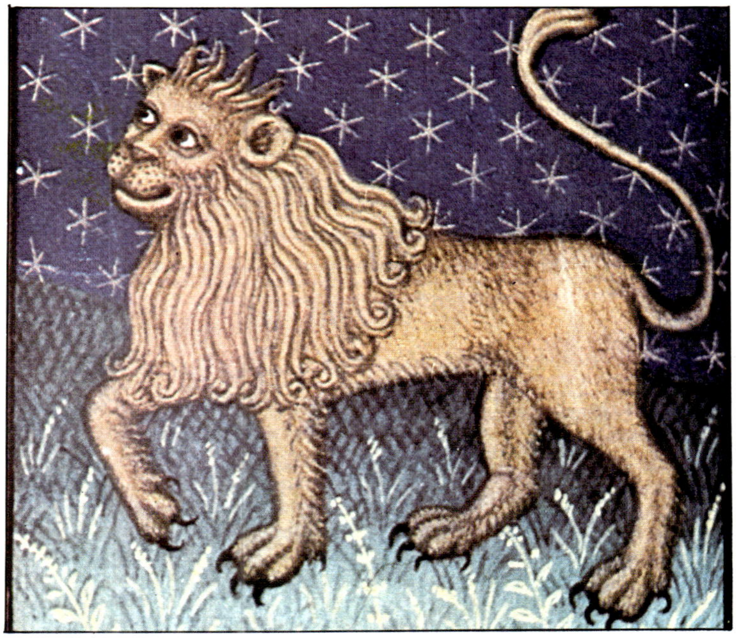

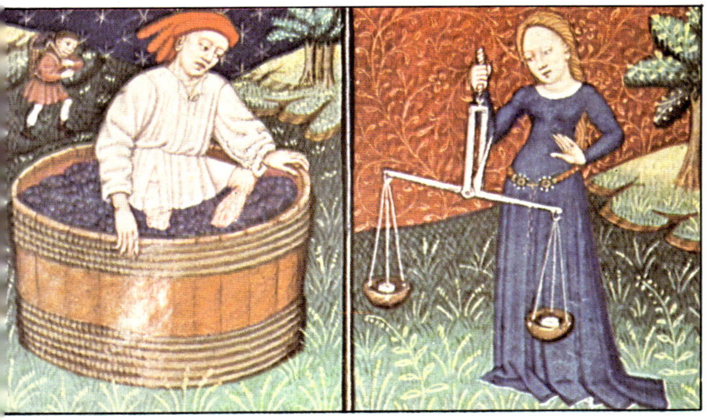

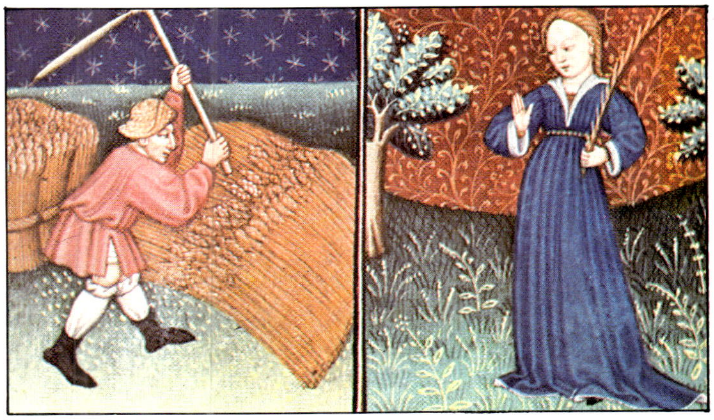

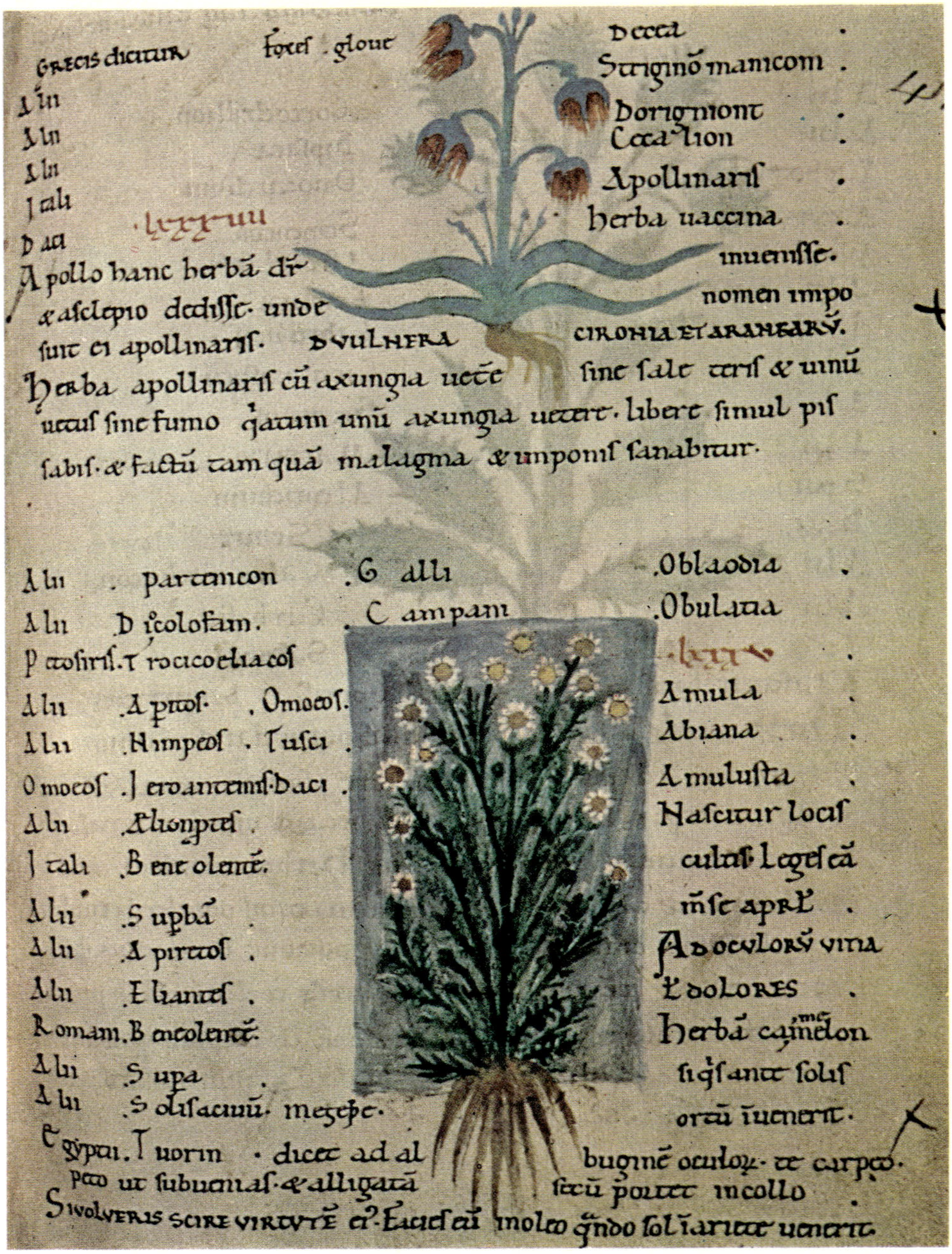

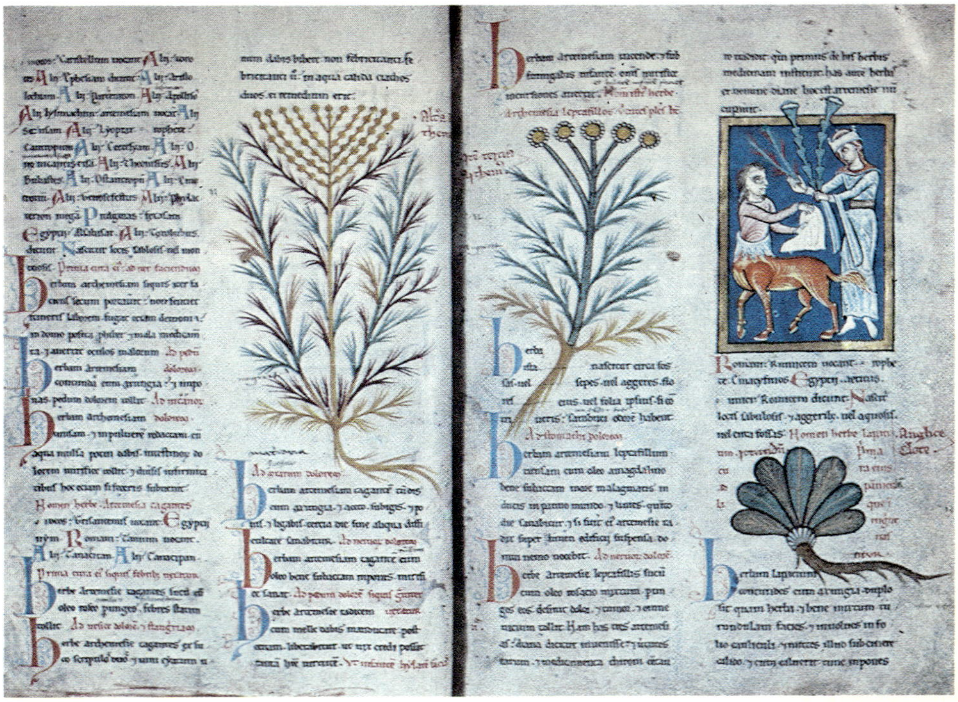

The manuscript pages of herbals are exquisite works of art in themselves. **Above right** *A herbal of the twelfth century illustrates two traditional healing plants. Above is the foxglove, which is still used in remedies for heart conditions; beneath is the camomile, which is still in popular use for making a soothing tea.* **Below right** *This thirteenth century manuscript shows the herb artemisia. The tiny inset represents the goddess Artemis handing the herb to the centaur Chiron, famous for his healing abilities.* **Opposite** *The frontispiece and some of the illustrations from Gerard's Herbal, published in 1597.*

Numerical power

Number has as much significance in folk remedies as the season or time of day; the seventh son of a seventh son has already been mentioned as a personage of unique worth in healing. A west of England cure is to bite the first fern seen in spring in a case of toothache (as with many other such recipes, success depends on toothache and spring occuring at the same time!) One and three, together with seven, are the favourite ritual numbers for the performance of curing tasks.

Multiples of three are also found, like this remedy for scalds and inflammations from Cornwall: Nine leaves of the bramble are moistened with spring water, and applied to the burned parts. While this is being done, for every bramble leaf the following charm is repeated three times: 'There came three angels out of the east; one brought fire and two brought frost; Out fire and in frost, In the name of the Father, Son, and Holy Ghost'.

Numerical charms today

If this seems a little far-fetched to modern readers what about the well-known cure for hiccups, drinking from the wrong side of a teacup? Not so long ago, the sufferer always spoke the following charm first, before stooping over the cup: 'Hiccup, hiccup, Rise up right up, Three drops in a cup are good for the hiccup.'

There the magical number three and ritual act are still present. And yet another survival from the days when number and date held so much influence is the rhyme about children's birth days:
'Monday's child is fair of face
Tuesday's child is full of grace' etc;

Modern students of psychology note the importance of ritual in successful curing: whenever we visit our local doctor, we pay great attention to the method he gives for taking his pills and potions. 'to be taken four times daily after meals'. Surely the exact following of these instructions is as important to us as the medication itself?

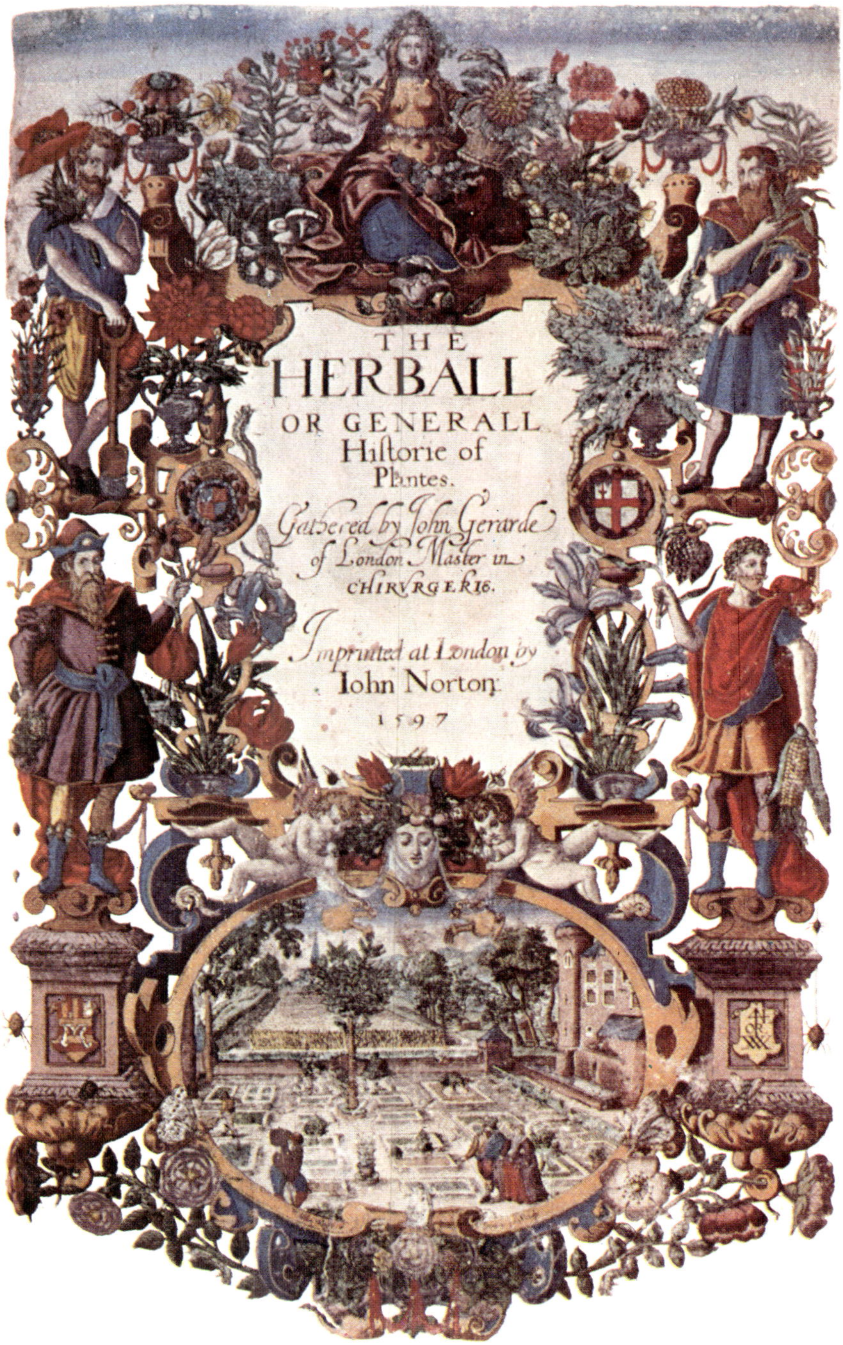

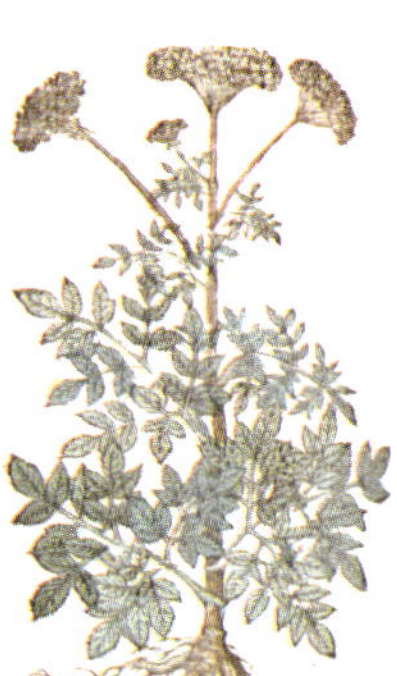
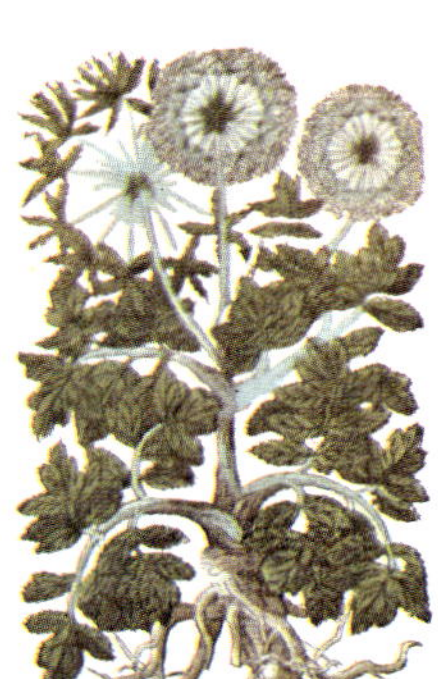
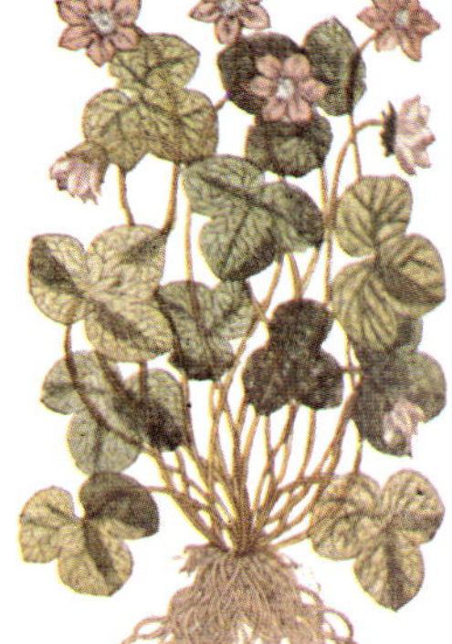
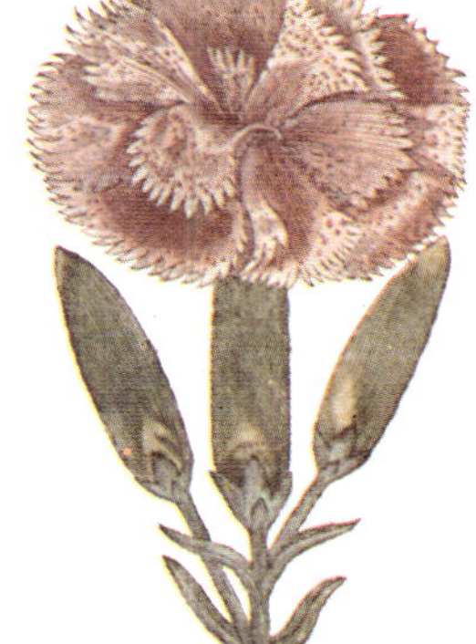
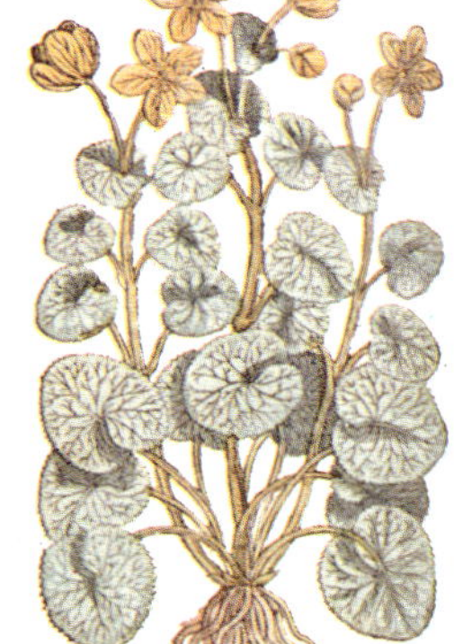

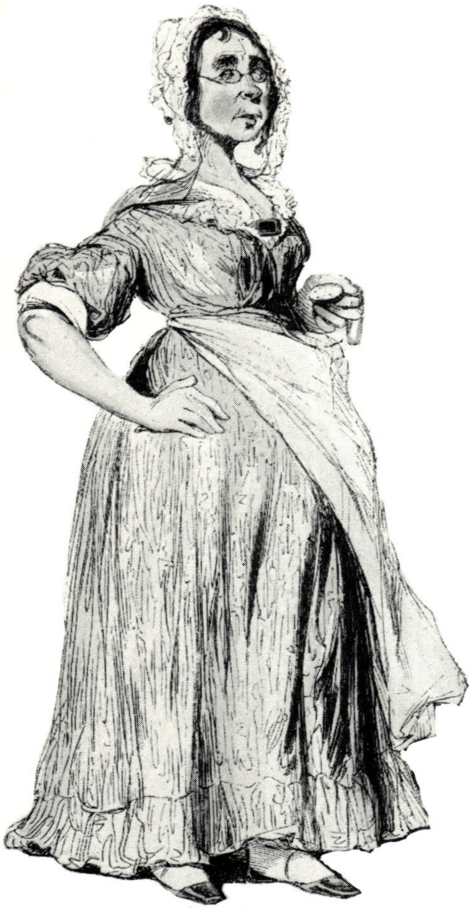

Above *The country midwife and* **Right** *The Irish fairy doctor are familiar figures in folk medicine. Their skills are based on years of experience, or sometimes on a healing gift which they themselves do not always understand.* **Below right** *Hospitals for the sick were often religious foundations.* **Opposite** *This fifteenth century Hebrew manuscript illustrates early medical teachings.*

Folk medicine versus quack medicine

While folk medicine has always confined itself to the treatment of short-term, fluctuating, or psychosomatic conditions, it should not be confused with 'quack medicine', where the mumbo-jumbo and the ritual masks a complete lack of feeling for the patient. Many practitioners of folk remedies, those who have 'the cure' in country communities, are people reluctant to use their powers, and they are often disdainful of money payments.

There are many bonesetters, massage specialists, or even mere touchers, who cannot understand quite why they have the gift, and treat it with respect, as a blessing to be shared with their neighbours. Herbalists and semi-skilled midwives are often greatly experienced in their field of practice, although their knowledge is based entirely on personal observation and years of working. In many countries of the world today, the two schools of medicine, the folk and the 'professional', work side by side, with mutual respect. This is the case in India, Africa, parts of Central and South America. In the western world, folk medicine survives only in herbalism, and much of the emotional need once satisfied by the traditional art is now absorbed into what is often termed 'fringe medicine', which is discussed in full later on.

Origins of quackery

Even 'quack medicine' finds a place in modern society, although its origins go back to the times when apothecaries and doctors were first emerging as scientific professionals. From the sixteenth century onwards, rules and regulations began to prescribe a doctor's or a chemist's training, and an inferior set of gentlemen, more concerned with profit than cures, offered the poor or the gullible some cheaper or more glamorous alternatives. Scientific medicine took well over 100 years to rid itself of the bat's wings,

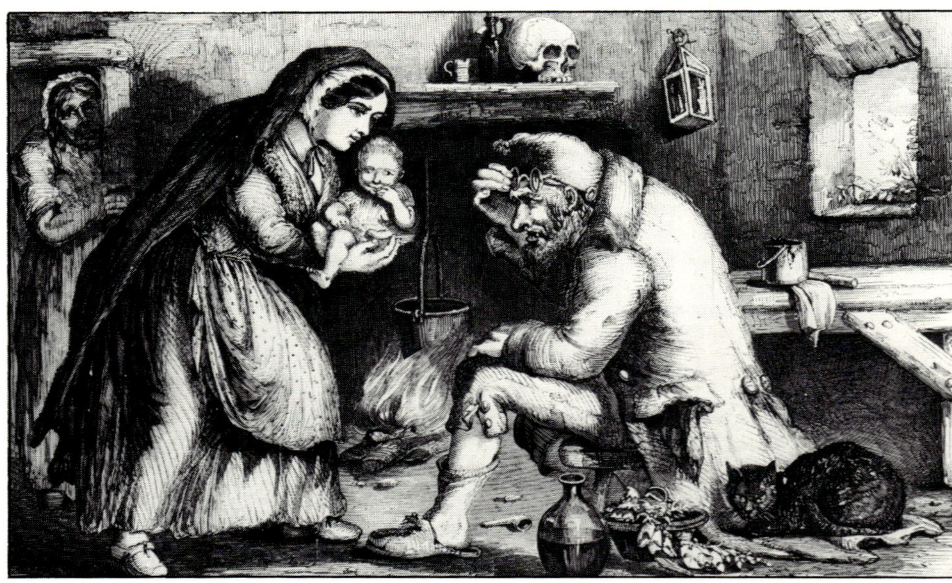

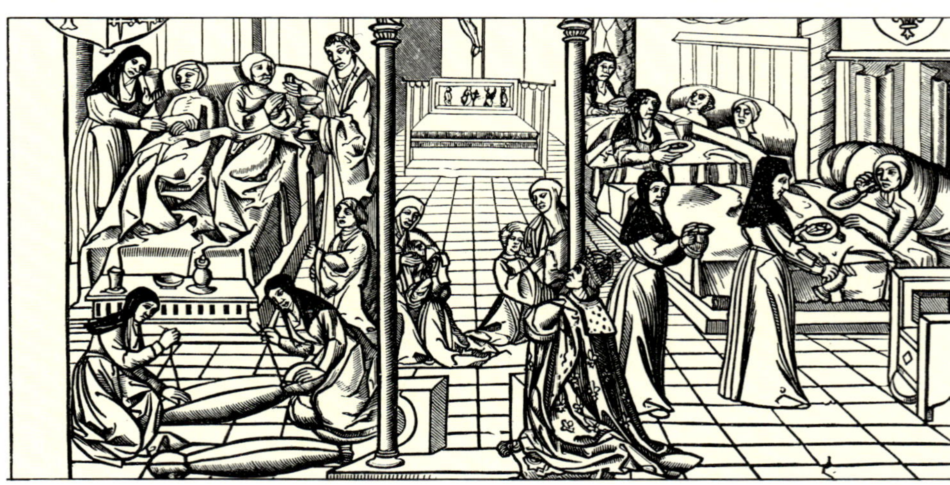

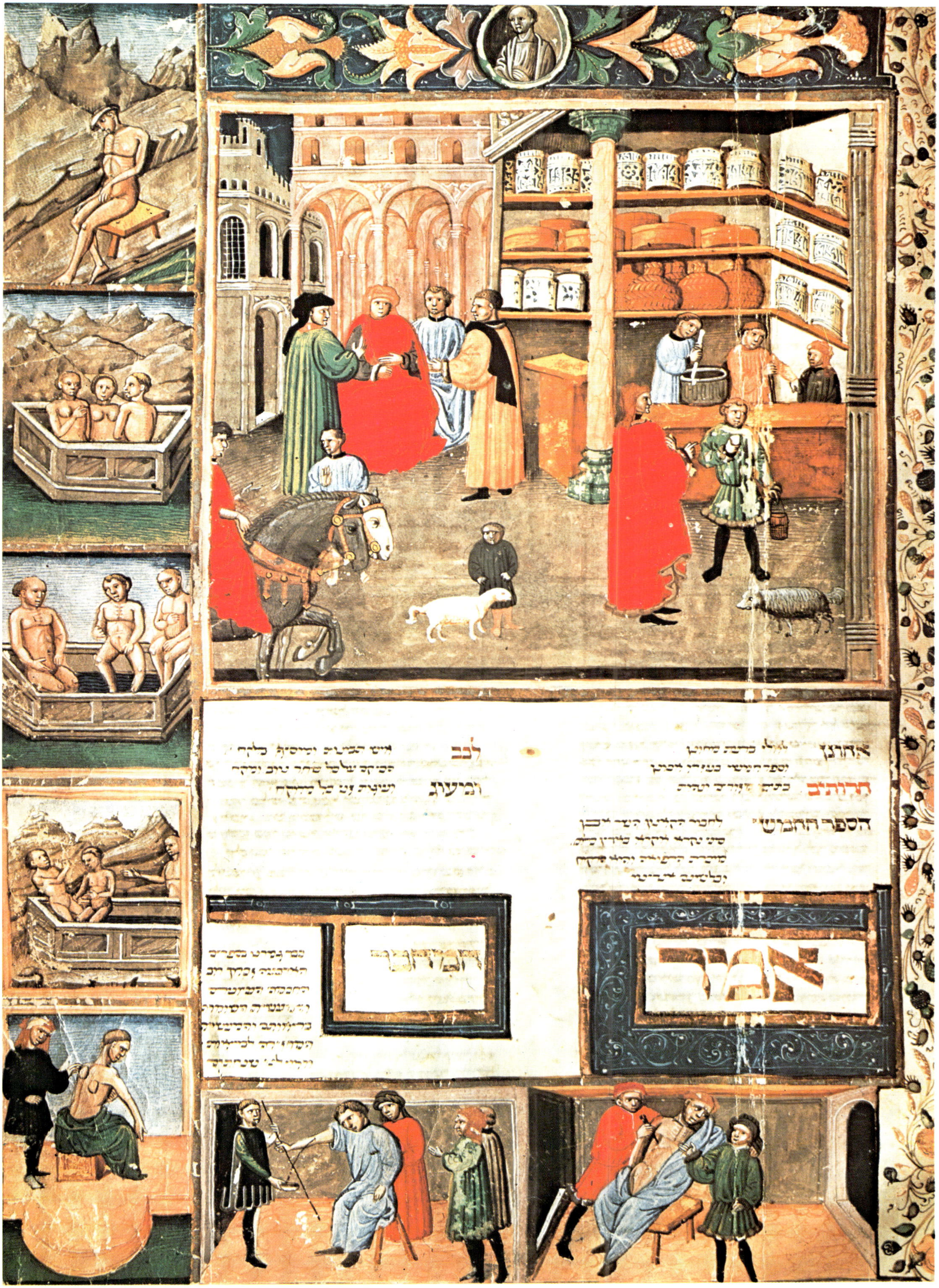
אמר

The othe of Hippocratus

I Sweare by Appollo the Physitian, by Æsculupius, by Higea, and Panacea: yea and I take to witnes all the Gods and Goddesses: that to my power I will uprightly observe this my othe: I will accompte my Maister which taught me this Arte, my father: his case hee shall command my life, and whatsoever he needeth I will give it him. As for his children I will hold his sonnes as my brethren, and if they desire the knowledge of this arte, I will teach it to them without stipent or covenant. I wille instruct my sonnes, and my maisters sonnes, yea and such as by hand wrighting are my scholars and sworn and adicted to Phisicke, the precepts, rules, and whatsoever else belongeth to the knowledge of the said profession, or touching the cure of diseases. I will appoint them to a diet, to my power; and in my judgement commodius. And I defend them from hurt and injury, neither shall the requests and petitions of any man, be they never so earnest, prevvaile with me to give poyson to any person to drinke, neither will I give my counsell or consent thereto in like manner I will refute the ministeration of any suppositorie, to the hurting or corrupting of the childe, in the time of my life. And in my profession I will shew myself pure, chast and holy. I will never cut any person that hath the stone, but will give place to stone-cutters, in the cure thereof, what house soever I come into, it shall be to the patient his profit. I will offer no injurie voluntarelie to anie man. I will eschew all wickednesse to my power, especially ye vice of Venerie, whether it bee my chaunce to deale with men or women, freedman or bondservant, whatsoever in any cure I shall see, heare or know, or in any other matter, yea though I bee not called to the cure myself, I will keepe it secret and unrevealed, so that silence therein be expedient. God graunt that as I trulie observe & keepe this my oath, I may have prosperous successe in my Arte and living. And according to the performance heereof, each man may sound my perpetuall praise. But if I transgress and break the same, I wish to God that in all my cures and other affaires I may have evil successe, and that everie one may discommend mee to the worldes ende toad's legs, mercury and quicksilver ingredients listed in its official pharmacopoeia. Quacks were unscrupulous.

Sir Kenelm Digby

An unscrupulous charlatan had only to turn to some of the old-fashioned remedy books, add one or two ingredients of his own, to come pretty close to orthodox medicines of his time. One of the most famous of all time, Sir Kenelm Digby, looked to Paracelsus, one of medicine's most magical philosophers, for his recipes. His first great success was a 'Sympathetic Powder', 'curing all green wounds that come within the compass of remedy', and 'prepared by Promethean fire', (1661). The Great Plague of 1665 was another incentive to quacks and charlatans, who peddled all sorts of ridiculous concoctions to the despairing citizens of London, like the 'Countess of Kent's Powder', made up of the black extremities of the feet of large sea crabs, pearls, coral, vipers, bezoar stones, plus a number of other significant folk-remedy ingredients used willy-nilly.

Tonics, Elixirs and Drops

A century later, patent remedies had achieved a new level of sophistication, with positively modern angles in advertising applied to them. 'Davy's Elixir' was one of the first, invented by a Leicestershire clergyman of the evangelical school, and bearing the now classic warning against 'cheap substitutes'. Each bottle announced that it was 'much recommended to the public by Dr King, physician to Charles II and the late learned ingenious Dr Radcliffe' (who needless to say never existed).

Another famous cure was Haarlem Oil, or Dutch Drops, still manufactured in Holland. First made in 1672, it was used as a preventive against all diseases. Some popular potions were more pleasing than harmful, like the delicious *Eau de Melisse des Carmes* dating from the same period – nothing more than a mixture of dried flowers, wine, and spices. It was a favourite cure for ladies' fainting fits, and a bottle stood handy on the mantlepiece of many an elegant parlour room. Its use was more social than medicinal.

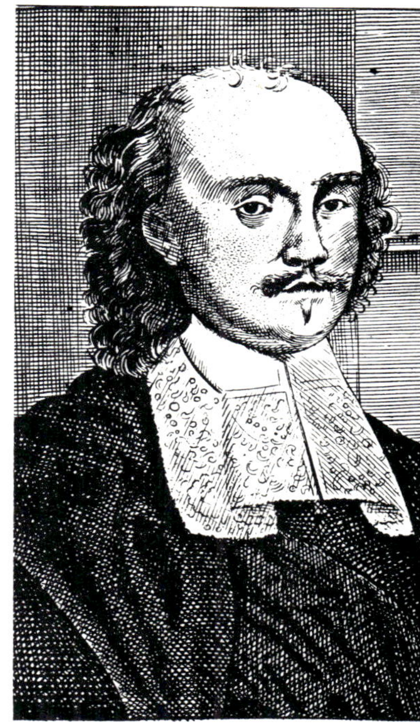

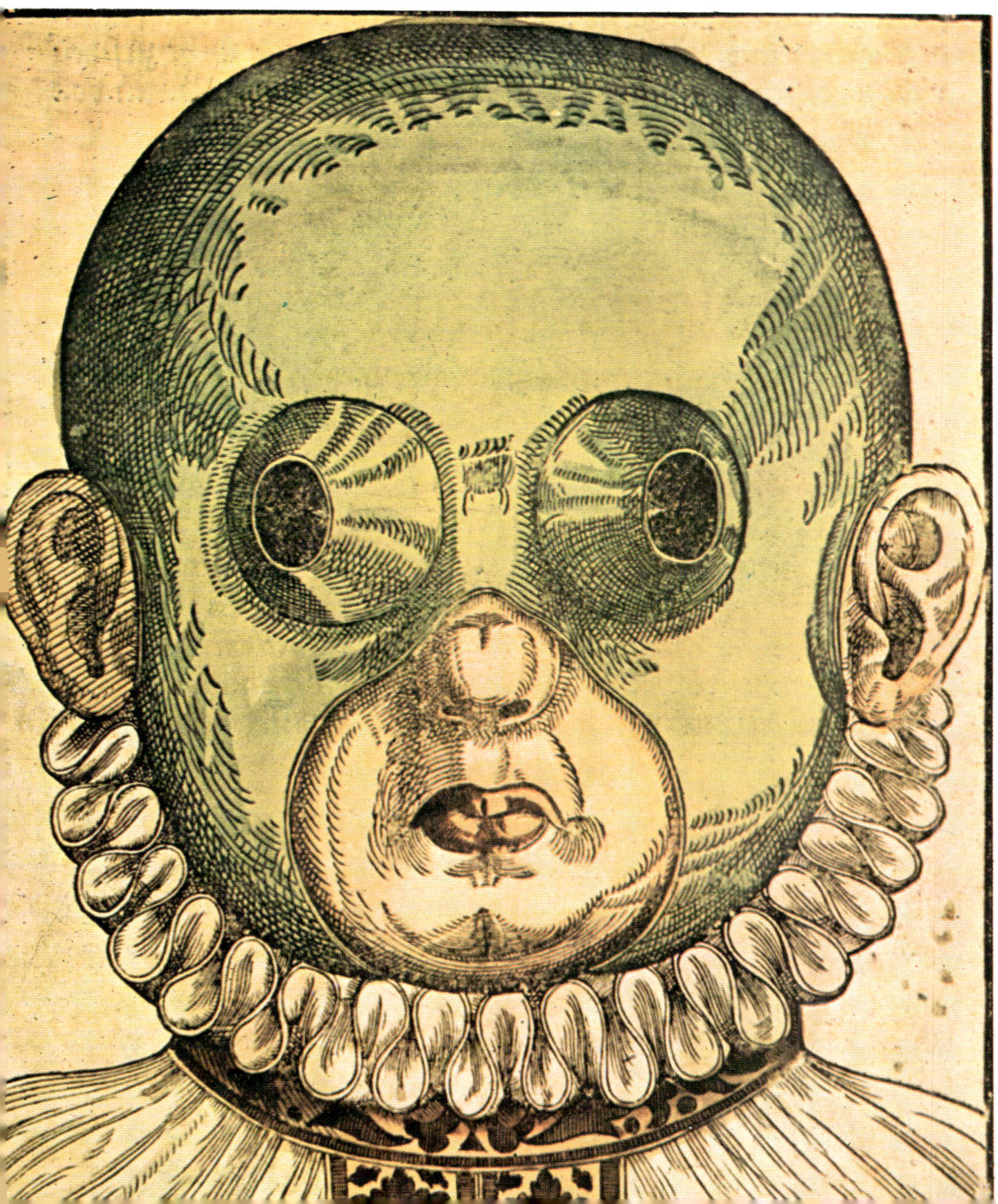

Above *Sir Kenelm Digby was one of the better known quacks of the seventeenth century.* **Below left** *This amazing device was invented by a sixteenth century oculist, and was used to correct squints. The same principle of covering up the stronger eye to force the weaker into activity is used today.* **Opposite** *A medieval translation of the Hippocratic Oath, which established a code of ethical medical conduct, and was first formulated in the fifth century B.C. by Hippocrates, the father of medicine.*

The gullible 1700's

The greatest period for quack remedies came with the 1700's when people had more money than sense, it seems. Spa towns rose in fashion, and cupping, bathing, and leeching assumed new importance in the array of bizarre treatments available to the weak-minded as well as the weak in body. High-living brought into popularity the *Eau Medicinale D'Husson*, to ease the inflammation of gout. Made of meadow saffron, it was first discovered by a British officer, and was made famous by the army. 'Godfrey's Cordial', a mixture of spices, opium, molasses, and alcohol, was another widely-admired tonic of the period.

This was an age when pseudo-science held a great charm for the gullible public. Any product with a suitably grand-sounding name could be relied upon to stir the fancy. 'Dr Bateman's Pectoral Drops', first sold in 1726 for 'rheumatism, afflictions of the stone, gravel agues, and hysterics', became a panacea in general consumption for over a hundred years. It travelled to America where doctors at the medical school in Philadelphia analyzed it in 1833, and found good cause for its calming effect. The main ingredients were opium and alcohol. Guaranteed to soothe indeed!

Another remedy with an impressive medical recommendation on the label was 'John Hooper's Female Pills' – of the best purging stomatick and anti-hysterick ingredients, duly proportioned.' Other best-selling mixtures of the eighteenth century include 'Dr James's Fever Powder', 'Betton's British Oil' ('extracted from the finest black, pitchy, flinty rock lying immediately over the coal in coal mines'), 'Frier's Drops', and 'Nathaniel Godbold's Vegetable Balsam', one of the first 'nutritional food supplements', many of which still find a huge market today.

Cures from the great frontiers

The nineteenth century remedies offered by quacks take on a positively international appeal, for many found their way to the frontier towns of the American West, or to the sheep farms of the Australian outback, while others made the journey in reverse, impressing pallid-skinned city dwellers in Europe with their efficacy because they were first used by strapping Red Indians or husky gold-diggers. All remedies of this sort are versions of sympathetic cures.

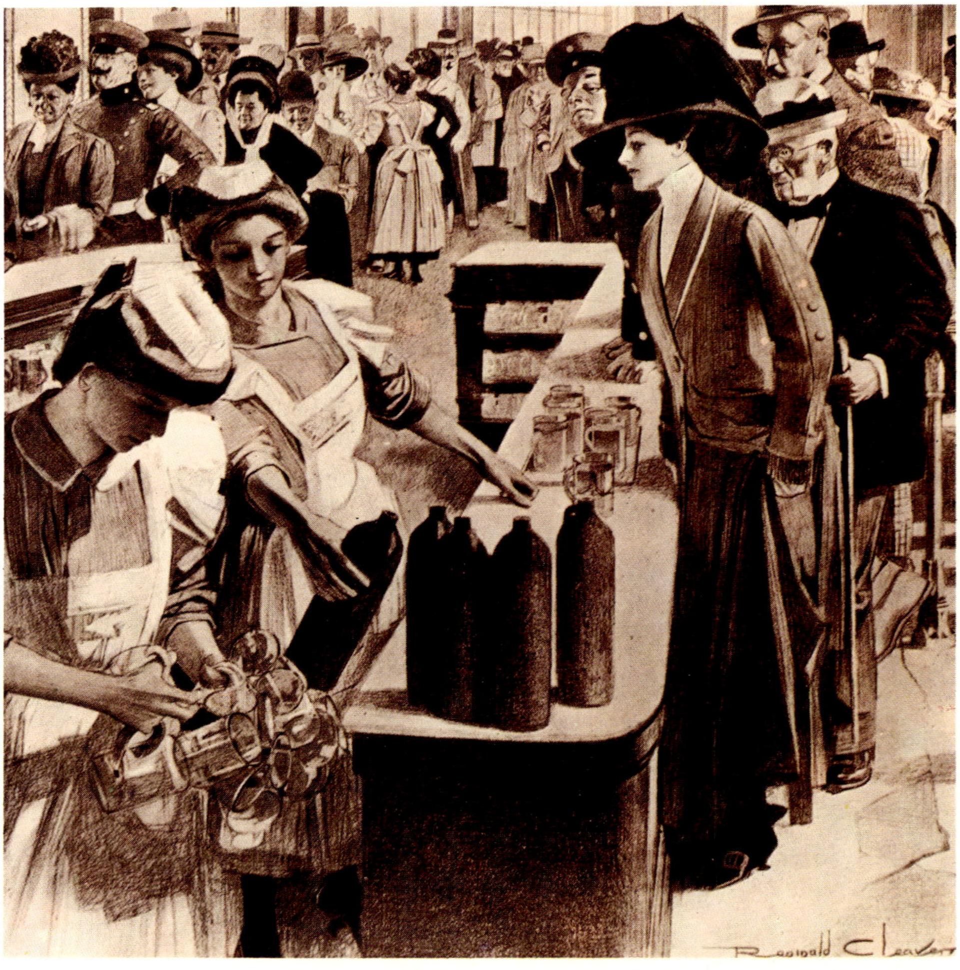

Right *For thousands of years, people have been unable to resist the belief that water from natural springs is a powerful cure for disease, despite the lack of evidence to prove it. Spas were particularly popular in the 1700's, and the fad promoted a brisk business in the sale of spring and spa water all over Europe. It has lasted up to the present.*

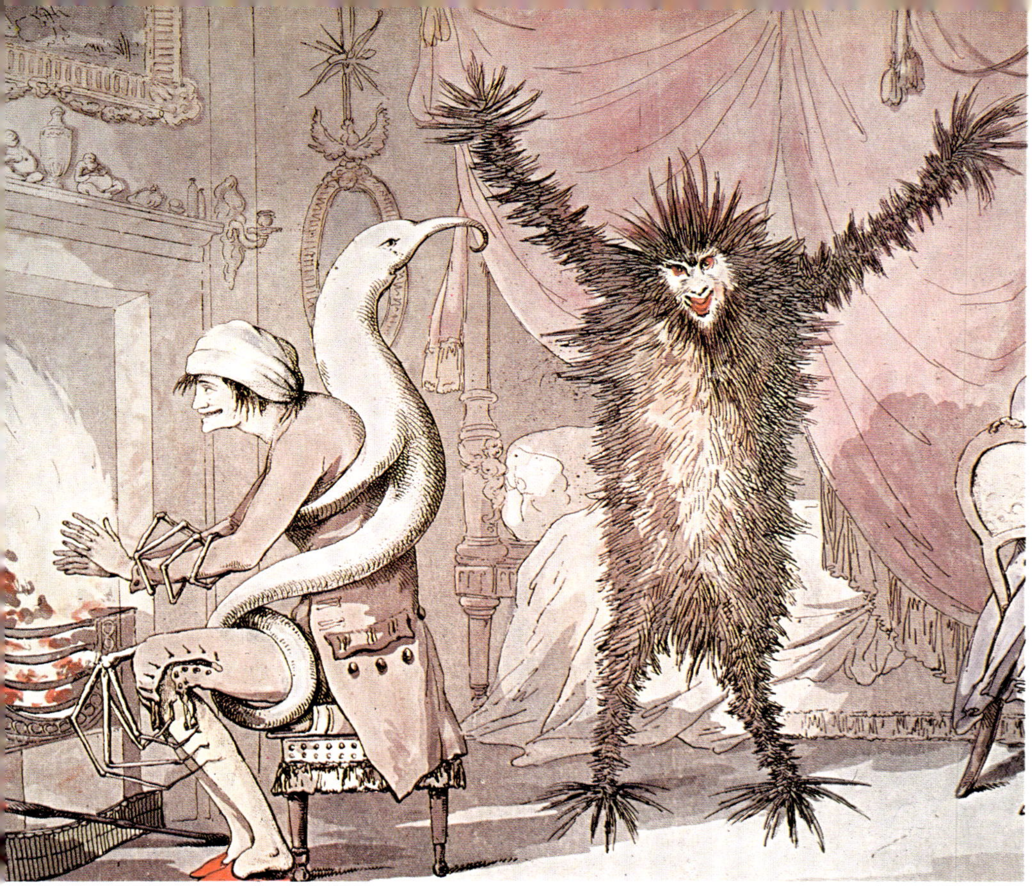

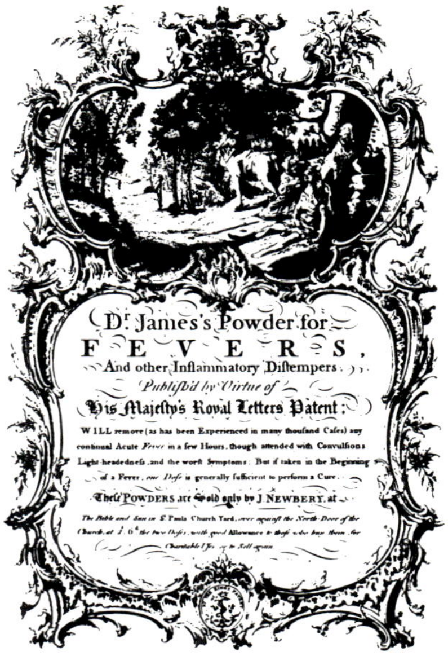

Above left *An eighteenth-century cartoon called 'Ague and Fever' by Thomas Rowlandson, depicts two stages of fever. The first stage is the ague, causing the sick man to shiver, while fever waits to pounce on him from behind.* **Above right** *An advertisement for the best-selling fever powders.* **Below left** *Edward Jenner discovered a method of vaccination for smallpox from a milkmaid who told him the country lore which said that someone who had already been infected with cowpox would not catch smallpox. The serum for the vaccine was extracted from infected cows, and Gilray's hilarious cartoon satirizes the innoculation by depicting cows leaping out of the patients' bodies.*

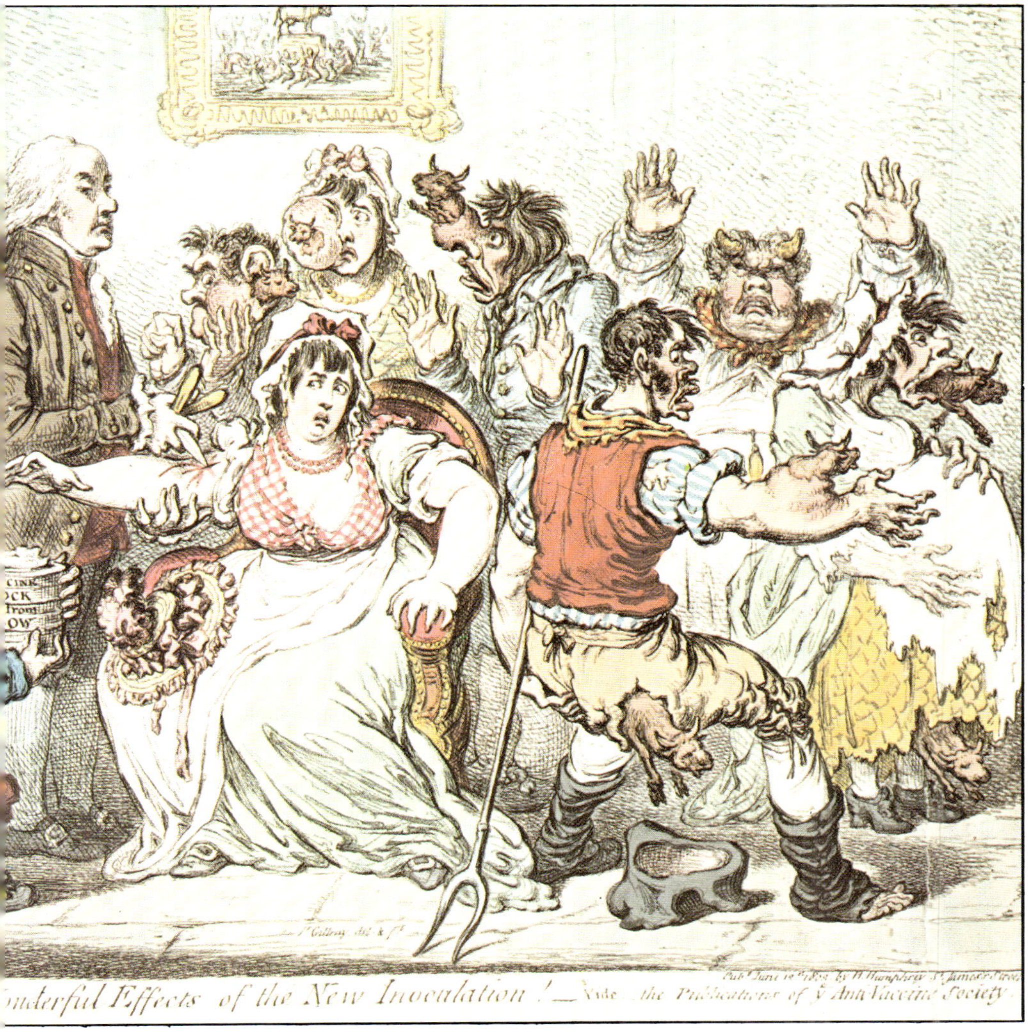

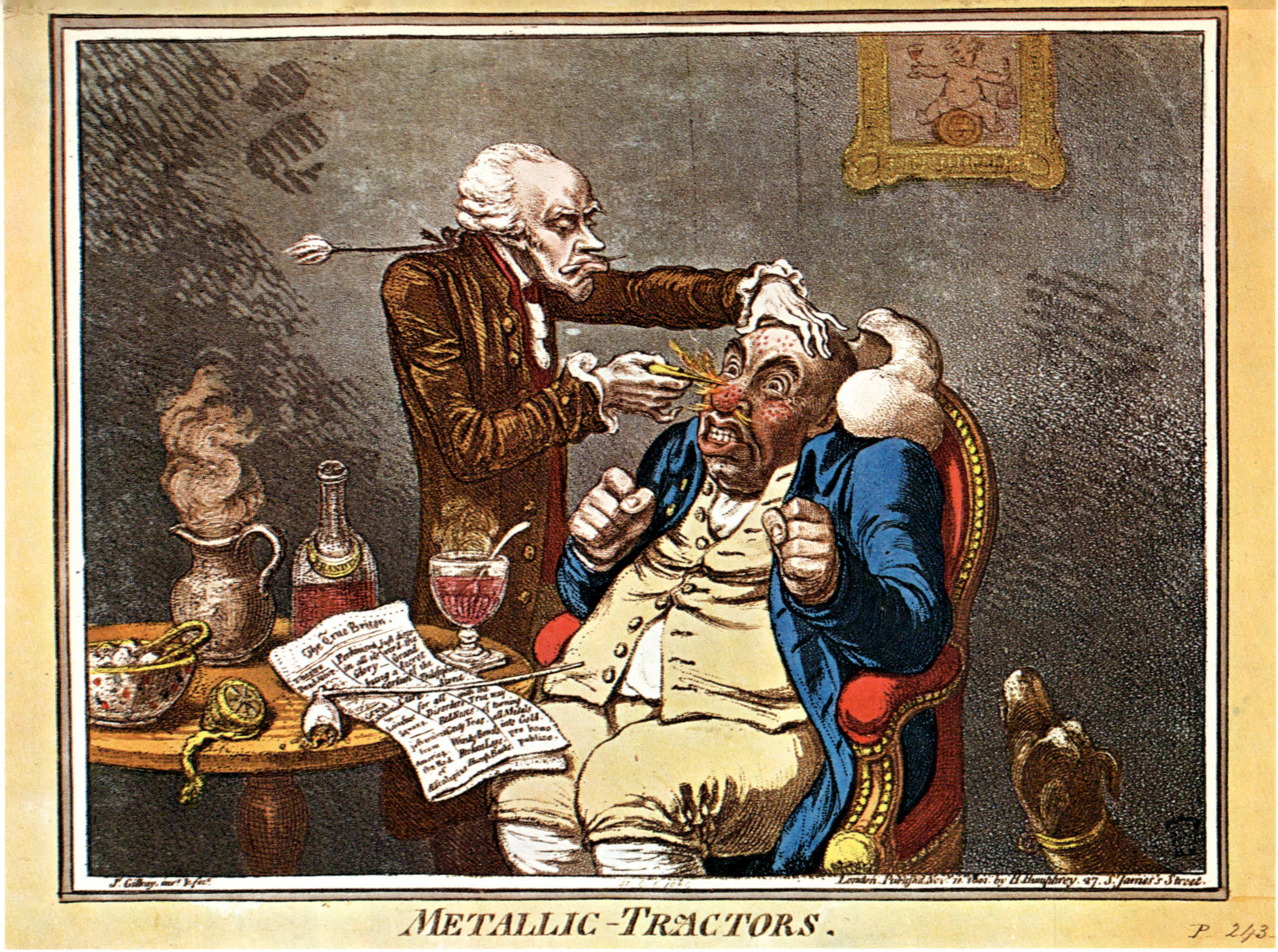

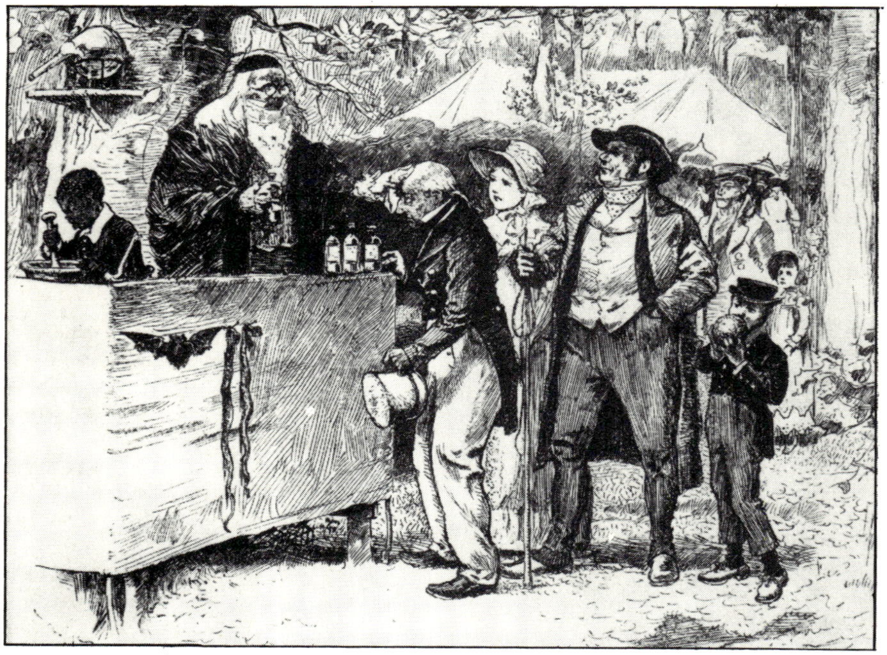

Above *An American quack of the eighteenth century, Dr Elisha Perkins, patented these electro-magnetic rods which were supposed to draw out diseases from the body.* **Below** *A Kentucky quack doctor selling his wares. They would be based on native plants.*

One of the most fearsome was the New World 'Drake Oil' or 'Indian Oil' that was highly popular in Western America and exported in large quantity to Australia too. It was merely hung in little bottles round the neck, and had reputedly been used by Indian tribespeople for hundreds of years, for rheumatism and a host of other aches and pains. (Indians traditionally used asafoetida bags in the same way, hung on a cord as a general preventive device.) 'Drake Oil' proved to be one of the wonders of the century: it derives its name from a Colonel E. L. Drake of Pennsylvania, the discoverer of nothing other than *kerosene* or paraffin. Once again, quacks had demonstrated their unfailing ability to latch on to anything new that will capture the imagination of the public, and convince them of a novel but powerful cure.

Medicines from America

America supplied some of the most long-standing patent medicines favoured by the nineteenth century, and indeed many of their names still sound authoritative and reliable. 'Dr Steers' Chemical Opodildoc', 'Ayer's Sarsaparilla', 'Paine's Celery Compound', 'Pinkham's Vegetable Compound' and 'Wright's Indian Vegetable Pills' are but a few of the most successful. One in particular, 'Perry Davis' Painkiller' received world-wide acclaim. It was a very versatile remedy, that could be used internally for all sorts of ills from dysentery to the common cold or stomach ache, or externally as a rub for sprains and bruises. It could even be

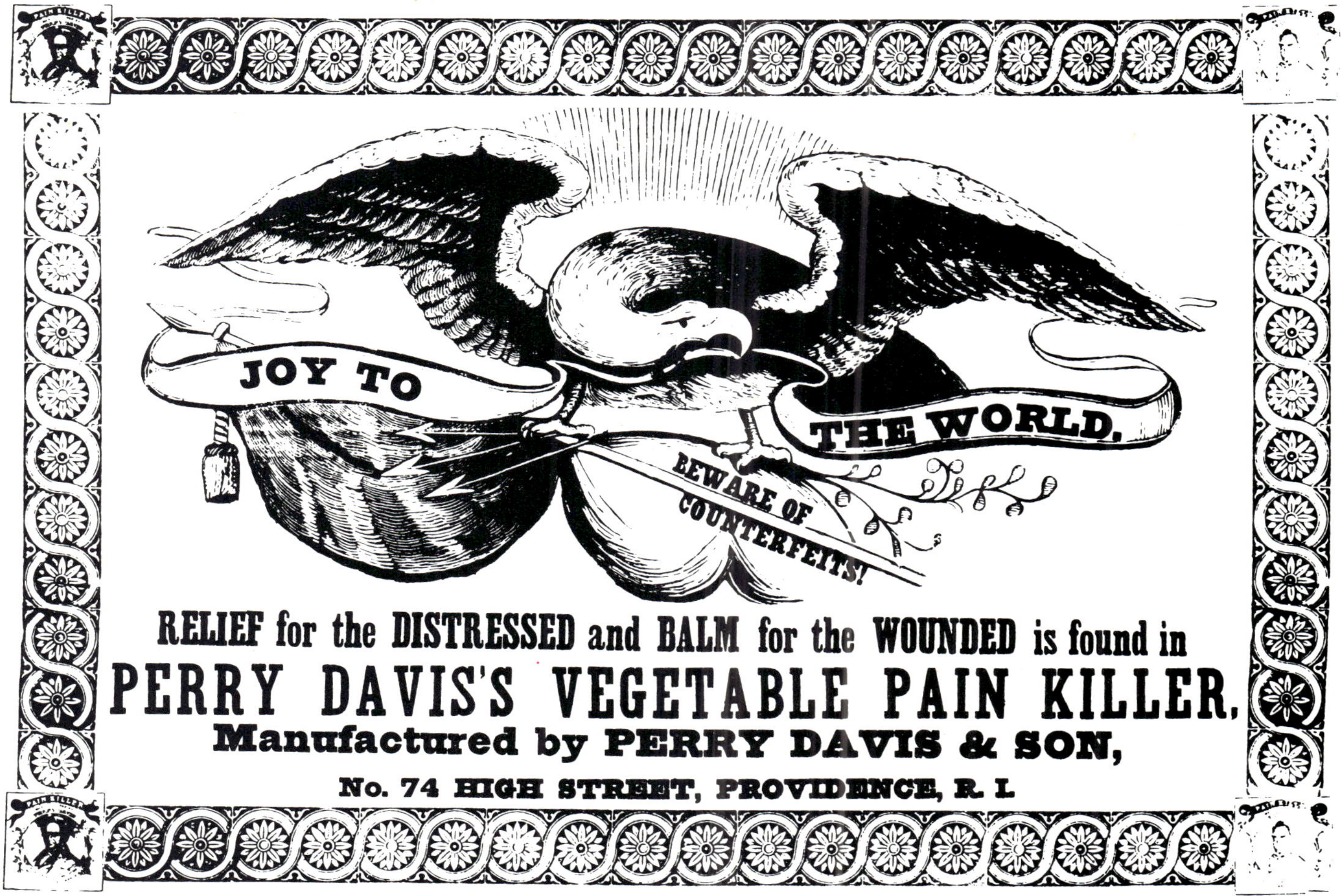

mixed with boiling water for colds, bronchitis, and other such complaints.

Sarsaparilla and sassafras were two New World substances that formed the basis of dozens of quack remedies, and both in fact have considerable value as curative agents. Sarsaparilla *(Aralia nudicaulis)* was originally used by many Indian tribes as a cough medicine; they crushed the roots and shook up the powder into a pleasing potion. American doctors found that the root has stimulant and sweat-inducing properties, and it was listed in the official US Pharmacopoiea from 1820 to 1882.

Sassafras, from a tree native to the North American continent, was another remedy much favoured by Indians of the eastern seaboard, and adopted by the settlers. It became a valuable export commodity from early colonial days, and achieved renown in Europe as a cure for colic, and the relief of venereal disease. Its traditional virtues are as a tonic, and sassafras tea is well-established folk remedy for high blood-pressure. Modern scientists isolate *safrole*, an aromatic oil from it, which is used as an antiseptic agent in dentistry, and still figures in the British Pharmacopoiea as a carminative and flavouring agent.

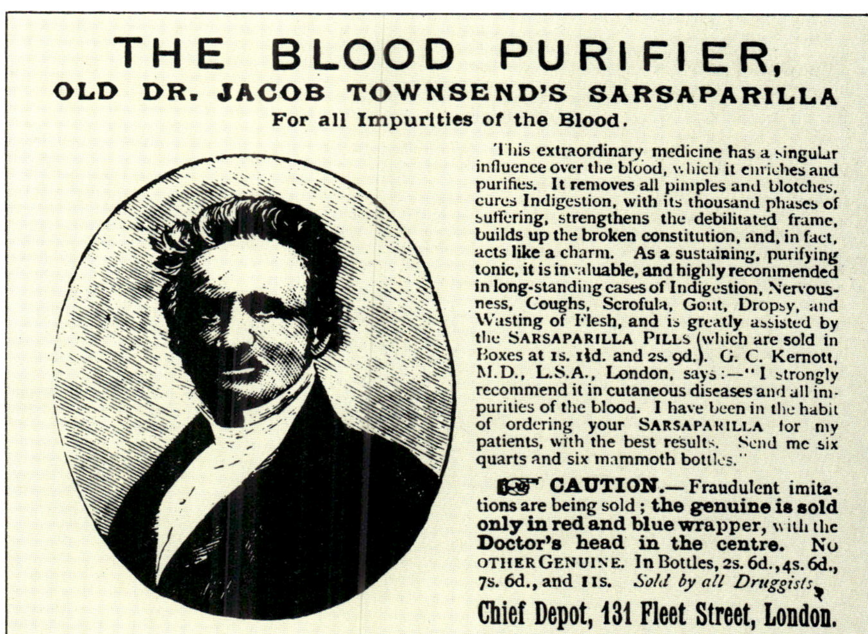

Patent medicines used today

Some of the better patent medicines still survive today, and there is no doubt that they contain simple but effective ingredients that make them at the least harmless, and often positively beneficial. Many mothers use 'croup waters' for that seemingly inexplicable painful crying

Above *The American eagle was often used as an advertising device, as with this popular patent remedy.* **Below** *Remedies such as this sarsparilla blood purifier originated in America. It was exported to England where it sold extensively.*

that babies endure in the early months. 'Dr Collis Browne's chlorodyne' is still marketed and 'Friar's Balsam' has achieved high respectability. The very age and familiarity of these remedies in part accounts for their success; once again, faith and confidence are essential ingredients in any cure. Many people resist new-fangled ideas, and prefer to stick to some tried and tested system of treatment which they trust, and have been handed down for years.

Fringe medicine

Quack medicines and patent cures still attempt to feed off the doubts and failures of orthodox medical treatment, but in the last few decades, a new phenomenon in healing has come about. There is a proliferation of 'alternative' or 'fringe' treatment, which claim that established methods are not only ineffective, but sometimes totally wrong. No quack would ever have set himself up in competition with a 'real' doctor, but sought always to mask his ignorance with respectability. Alternative medical practitioners, while careful not to make claims that can be refuted by orthodox doctors, nevertheless believe very firmly that they are offering something as good, if not better, for particular kinds of suffering. In this way, fringe medicine is taking over the place occupied by folk medicine in history. The essential ingredient in the relationship between healer and patient is one of trust and confidence, and each system of fringe medicine offers just as elaborate a logic or system of explanation as the old folk remedies used to provide.

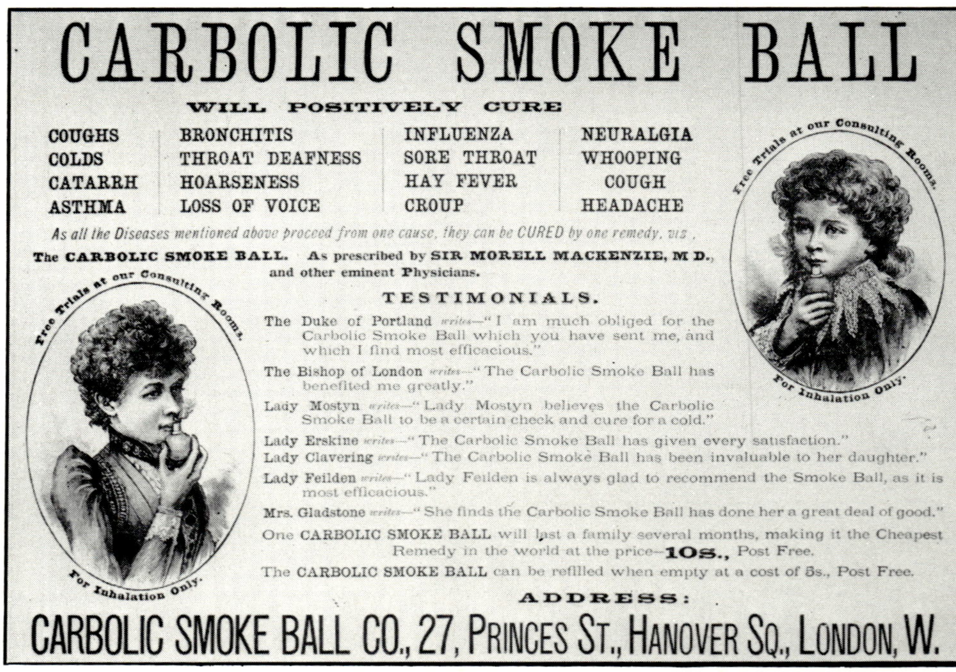

Right *Remedies claiming to cure a multitude of illnesses were frequently patented as is demonstrated by this advertisement for a 'carbolic smoke ball'. Also very common was the use of important personages whose names were used to back up the claims of the medicines.* **Below** *One of the fringe treatments today uses 'music therapy', but the idea is ancient. This fourteenth-century illustration from a medical book shows music being played to relax a patient in surgery.* **Opposite** *A Victorian quack peddles his wares in a poor urban street.*

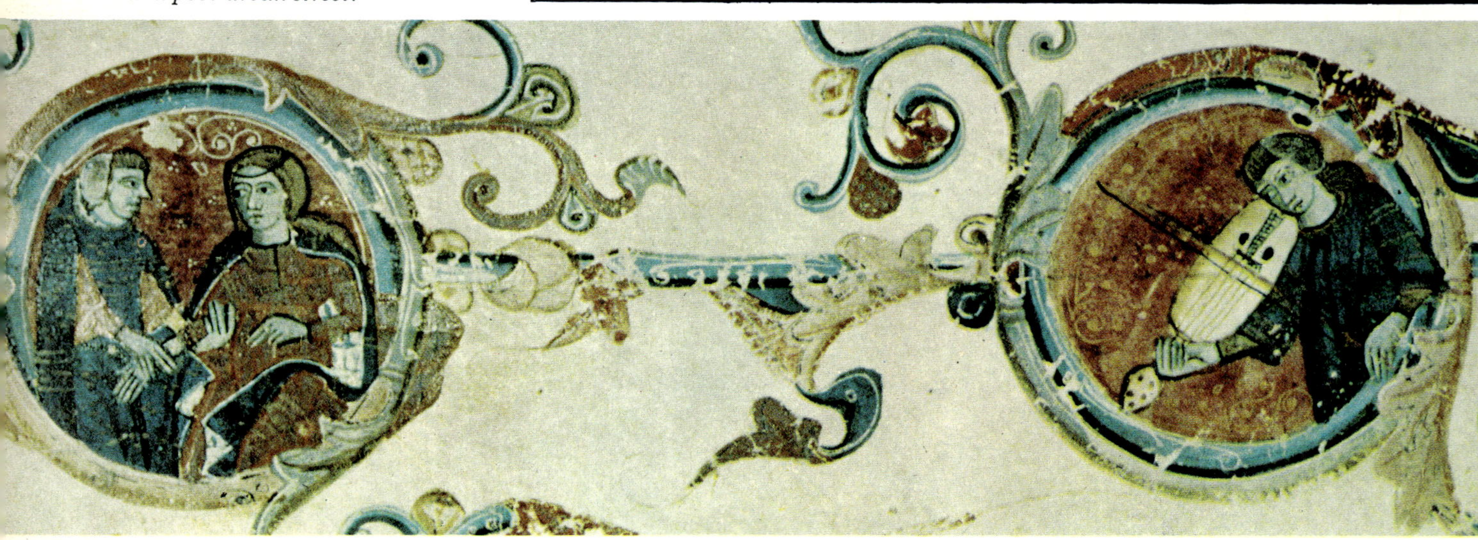

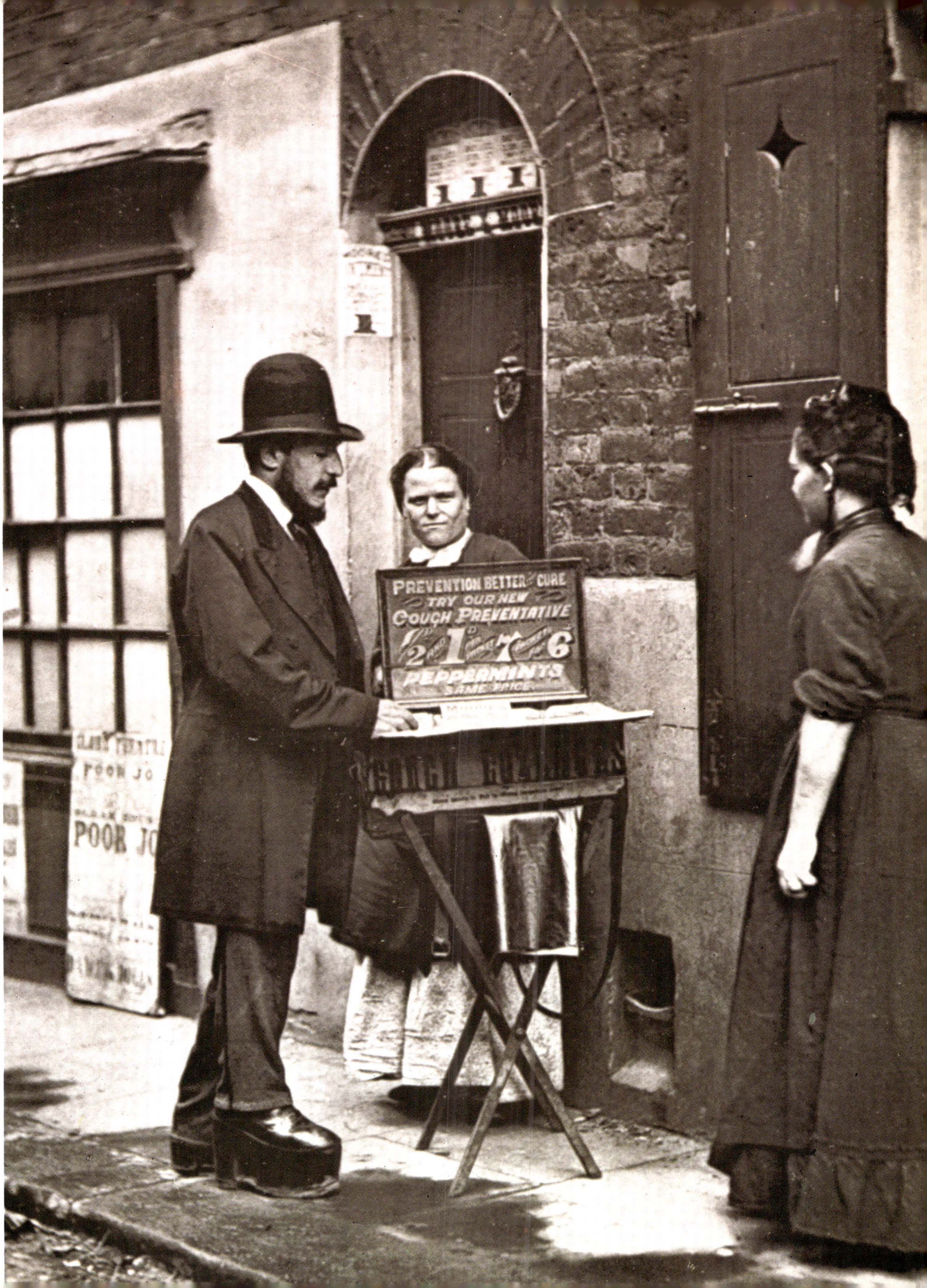
PREVENTION BETTER CURE
TRY OUR NEW
COUGH PREVENTATIVE
1D
7
6
PEPPERMINTS
SAME PRICE
POOR JO
POOR JO

手少陽三焦經之圖

凡二十三穴
左右共四十六穴

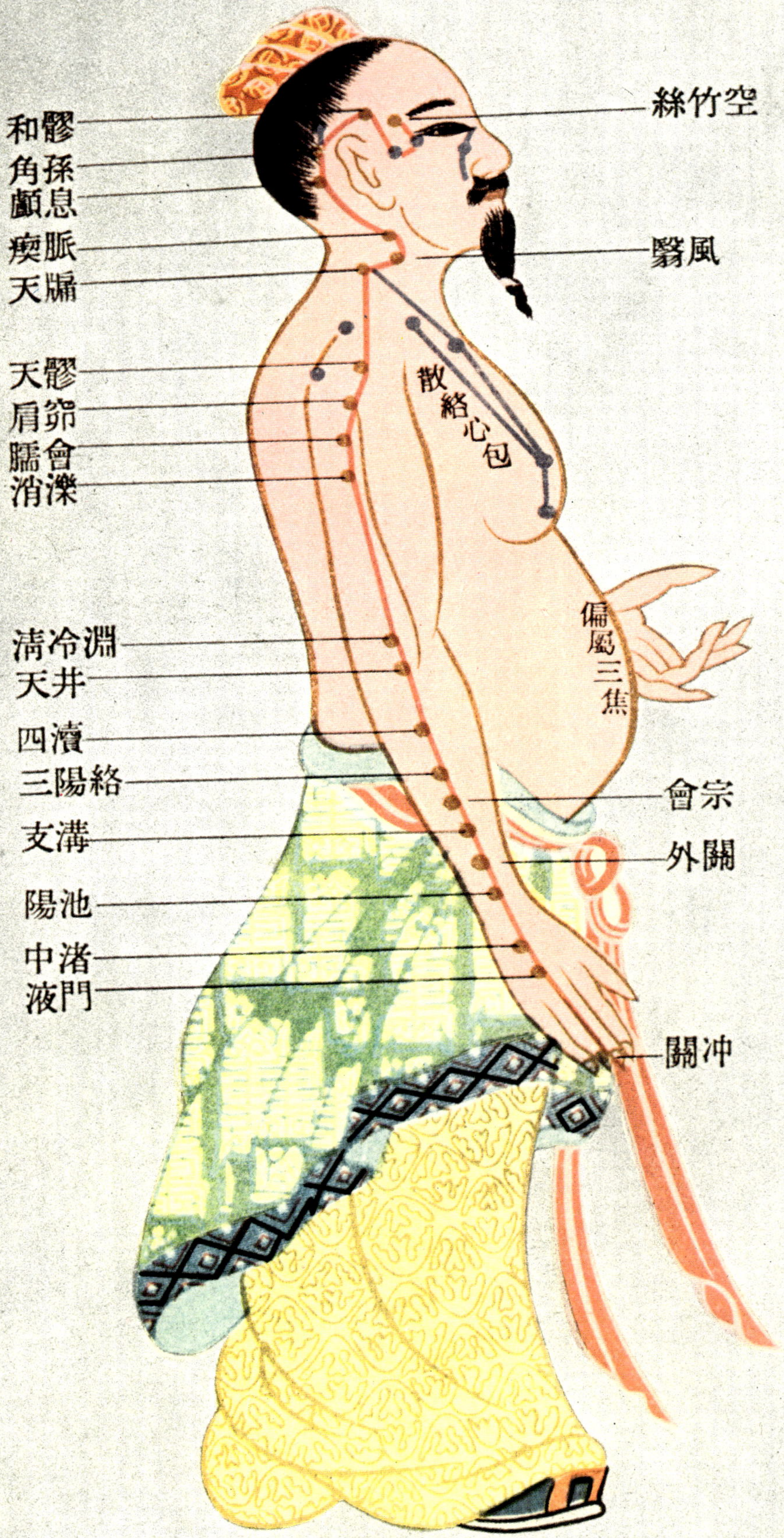

圖五十七——仿明版古圖(三)

Acupuncture

In fact, certain branches of fringe medicine are really folk-medical methods from other countries, with just as long a tradition as other favourites like herbalism. Currently most popular is the Chinese art of acupuncture, an extremely complex system of treatment whereby fine needle points are stuck into selected spots on the body in order to cure a disorder or imbalance in some other portion of the anatomy. The basic idea behind acupuncture is that there are 'channels' or 'meridians' in the body, through which energy flows. When a person is sick, the flow in the appropriate channel if affected, possibly some distance away from the site of the original upset of the body's balance. If the fine needles or more correctly, small lances are inserted at very precisely located spots on the meridian or channels, then the resulting stimulation to the whole body can produce a cure.

The acupuncture controversy

What baffles modern science is that there is no apparent explanation for improvements so achieved by acupuncture, although it has to be admitted that successes often occur. A particular area of doubtfulness surrounds the selection of the place for the insertion of the needle; skilled practitioners seem to know where to do it by pure guess work or intuition, which makes scientific analysis and approval very difficult.

Statistics from Communist China, where acupuncture is a respected and widely-used form of treatment, show a remarkably broad coverage of illnesses with it: malaria, enteritis, dysentery, bronchitis, arthritis, tonsilitis, nervous stomach upsets, influenza, rheumatic diseases, cholera, edema, epilepsy and infantile paralysis. A success rate of 92.3 per cent is reported for the treatment of appendicitis, and many surgical operations are performed without the need of anaesthetics. In this country, however, acupuncture is not used for so many types of illnesses, although it has proved helpful in cases of rheumatism, arthritis, and other forms of muscular pain. The difficulty in its recognition here is that in its true form, as practised by the oriental doctors, it is a preventive measure, whereas in the west people tend to try it out when all else has failed. Its value is still hard to assess.

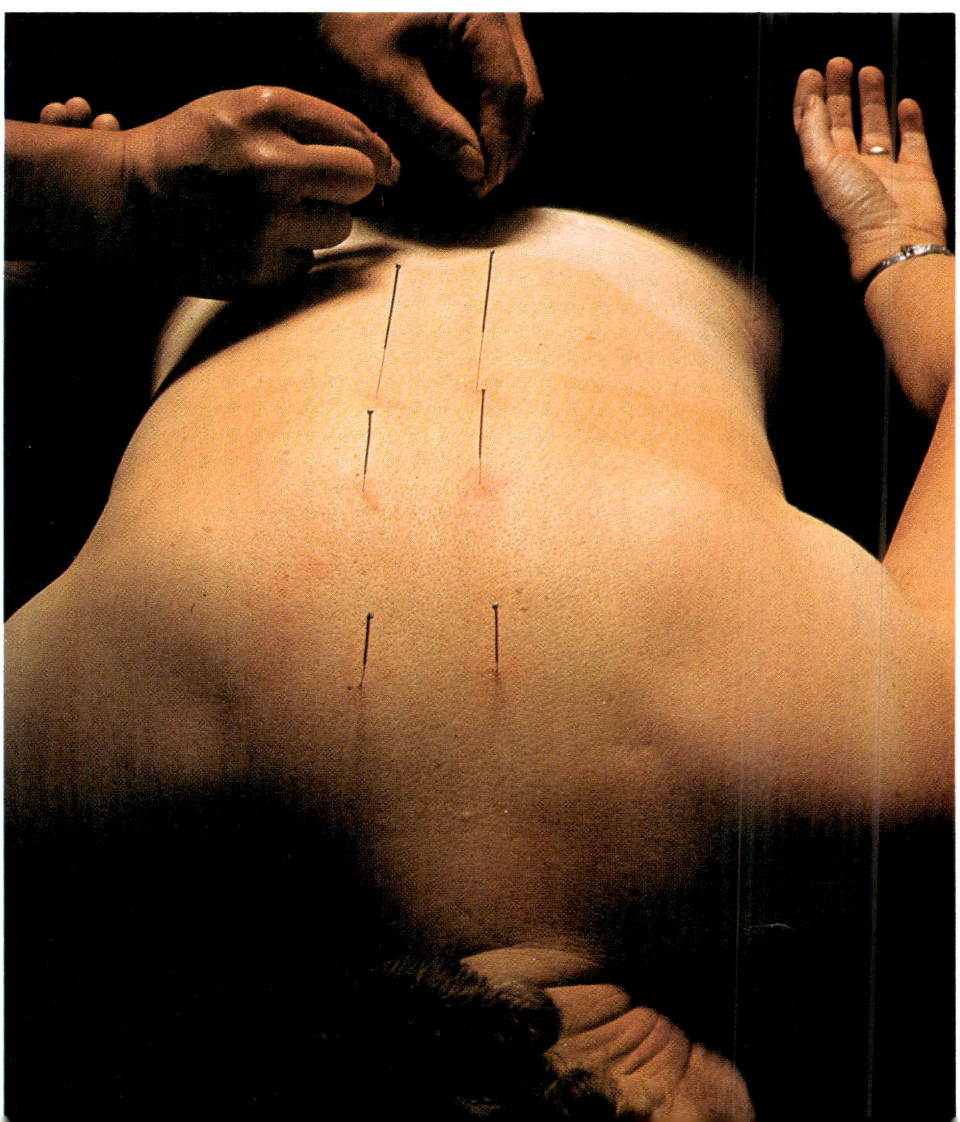

Opposite *Chinese acupuncture is a healing technique whereby fine needles or lances are inserted into key spots on the skin to keep the body's life-forces in harmony. Chinese charts provide only a rough guide to these points, and it is experience which really provides results.* **Left** *A close-up of the needles being inserted. Though great claims are made in China for the efficacy of acupuncture, western doctors are still sceptical.*

Extreme right *A dramatic close-up of an ornate jar used for storing homeopathic substances, in this case,* arnica. **Above centre** *A homeopathic dispensary, and* **Below centre** *huge storage jars.* **Below** *The founder of homeopathy, Samuel Hahnemann.* **Bottom** *A contemporary engraving of the London Homeopathic Hospital founded in 1849 by Frederick Quin.*

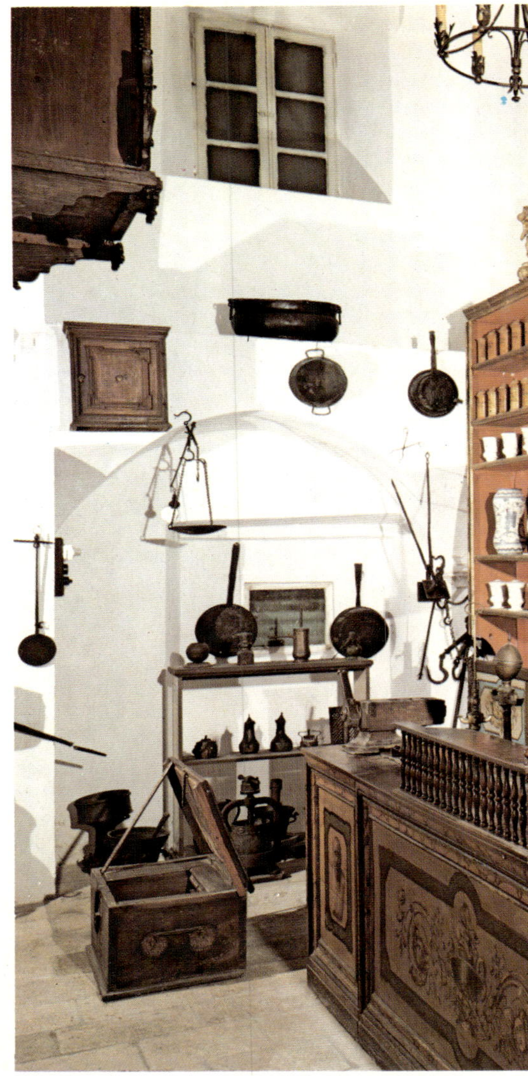

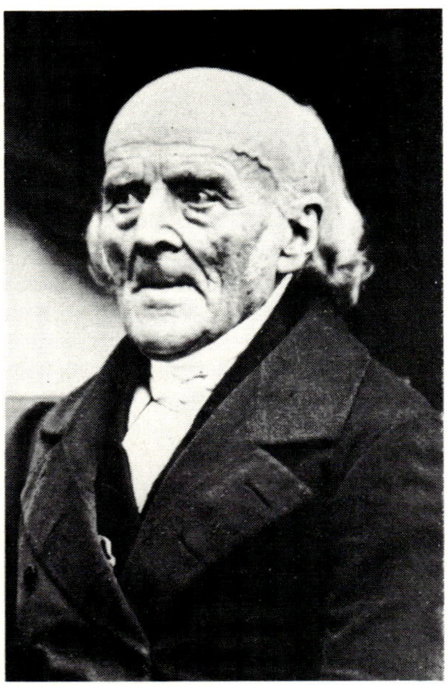

Homeopathy

Homeopathy has been a popular alternative treatment system in the west for considerably longer than acupuncture; a hospital specializing in its use was established in Soho, London, in 1850. The founder of homeopathy was Samuel Hahnemann, a distinguished doctor in Saxony in the late 1700's who formulated the theory that 'likes should be treated by likes' – not with complicated potions made up of dozens of ingredients, but with one simple, powerful drug.

He stumbled upon his theory when testing *cinchona*, the Peruvian bark that yields quinine. It gave him a fever, though of course he well knew that quinine *cures* fever too. He believed that the drug set up its own fever in the body, that counteracted the effects of the one causing the illness. His ideas were modified by another physician, Sydenham, who saw not a battle or conflict between the two activities, the work of the illness and the work of the curing drug, but more that the body itself puts up a fever as a defense against the attacking illness. So, if a drug which induced a fever was administered to a patient, it helped him to put up his own bodily battle against the intruding disease.

The small dose theory

Hahnemann continued his work with drugs using gradually smaller and smaller doses on healthy people to see what effects they produced, then giving that same dose to a patient suffering from a similar set of symptoms as the drug itself induced. In a way, he wanted to use drugs to work a cure from the inside out, rather than bombarding the body with a massive 'counter-dose', which seemed to be the policy behind orthodox medicines,

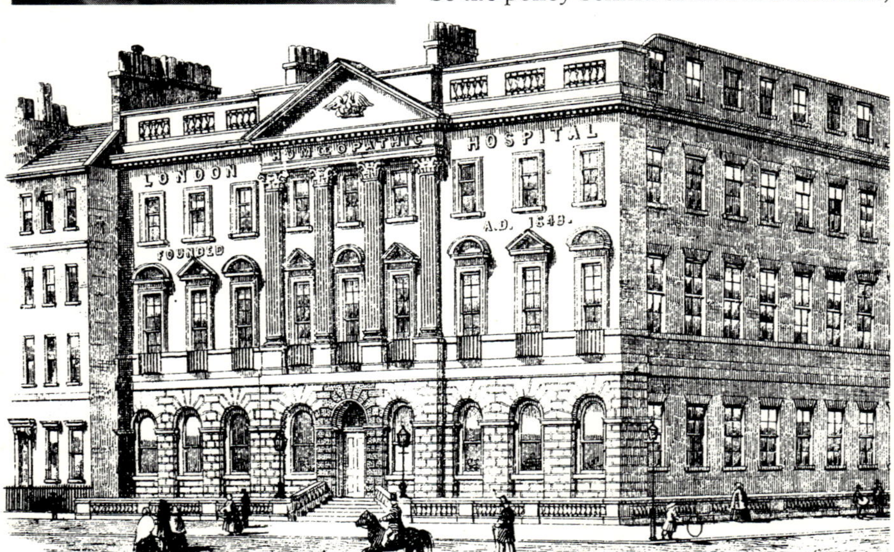

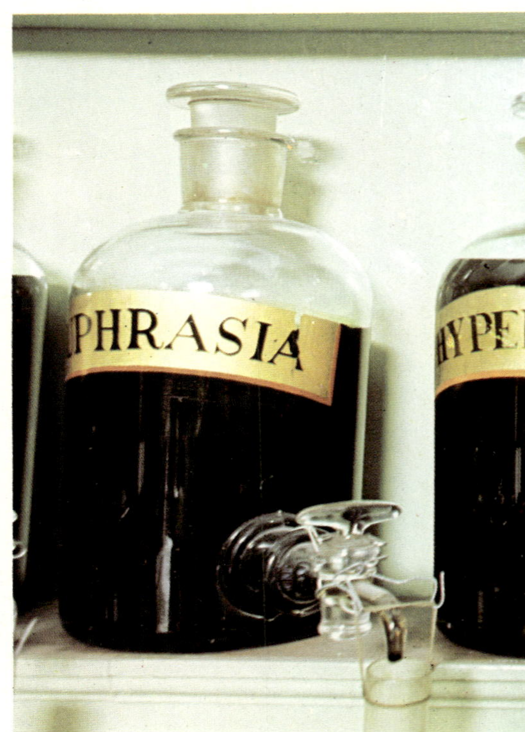

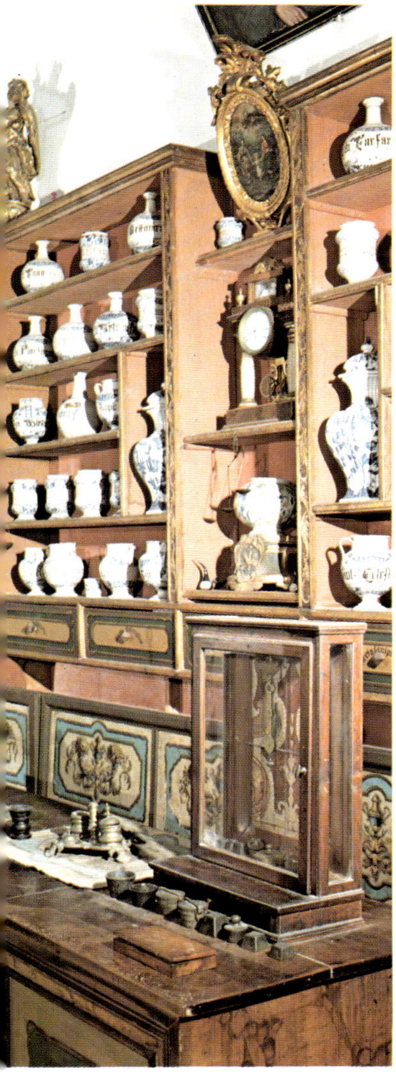

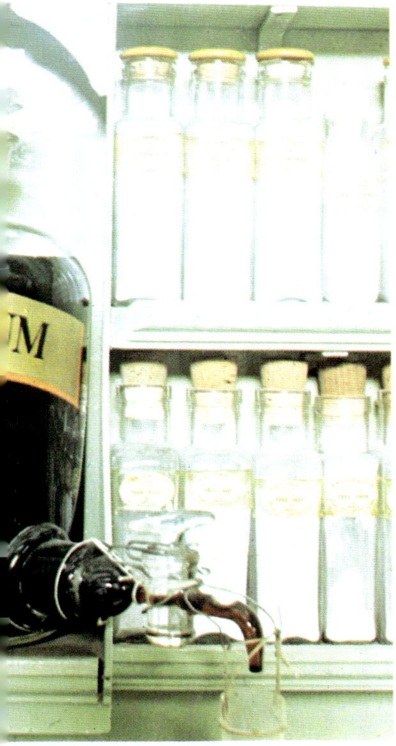

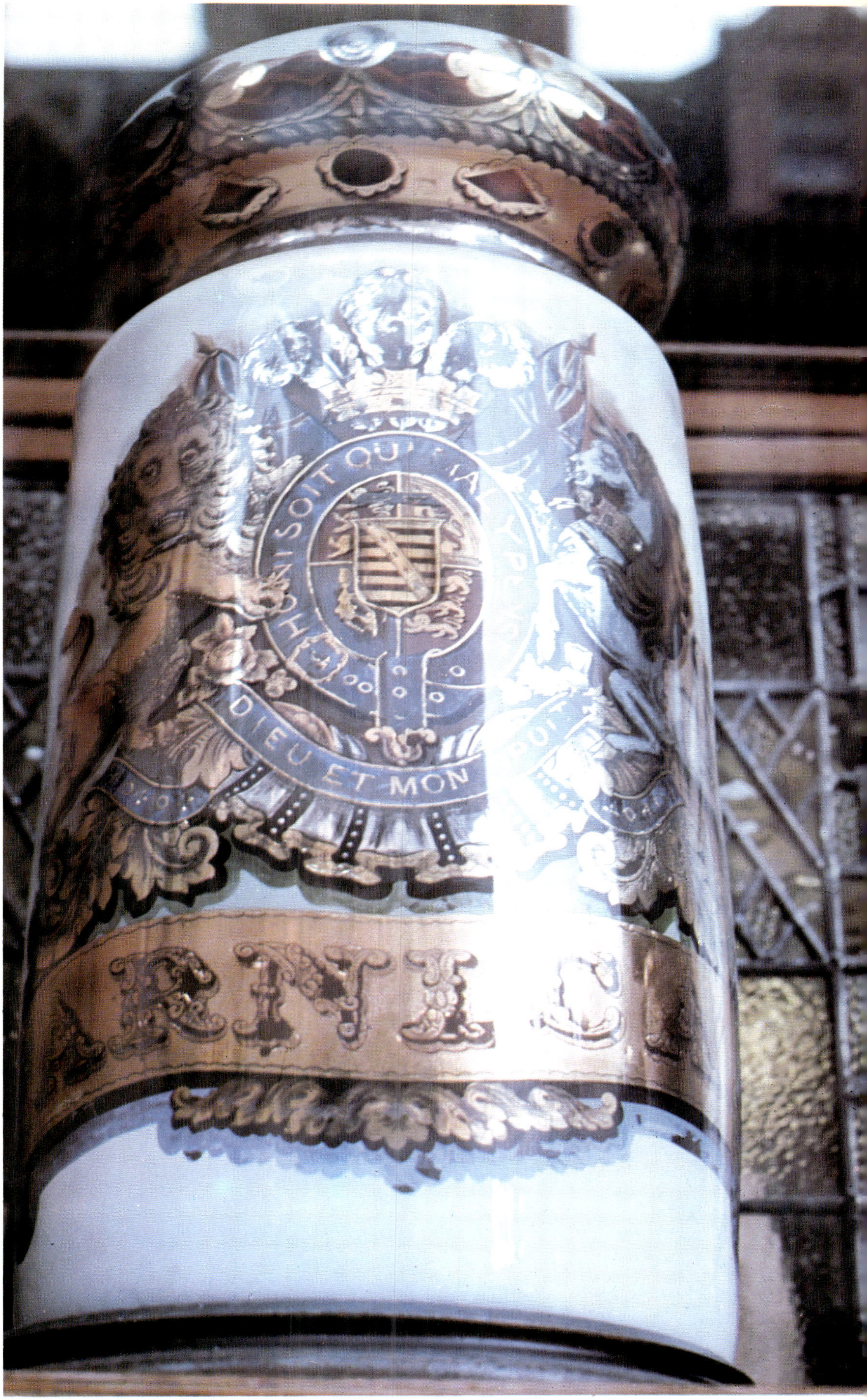
DIEU ET MON

Right *Frederick Quin, founder of the original homeopathic hospital in London, had studied under Hahnemann. He attracted many distinguished followers, including members of the royal family. The present Queen, Elizabeth II, has a homeopathic doctor among her physicians, and her father named one of his racehorses* Hypericum *after a homeopathic remedy.* **Below** *Porcelain storage jars used in homeopathy.*

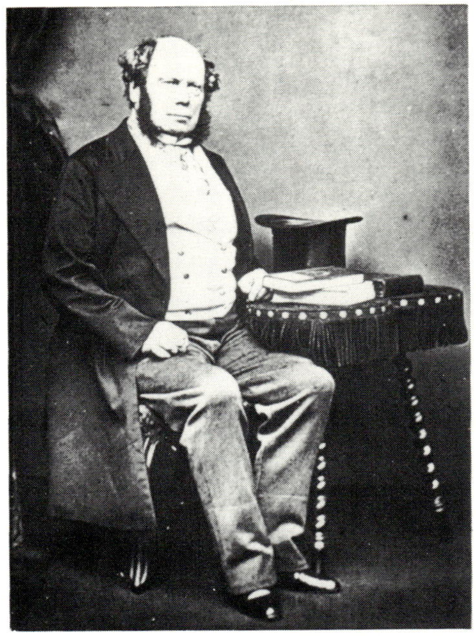

'From the inside out' also meant that for the first time, great attention was paid to the individual patient's background, habits, circumstances and general bodily experience, so that the drugs administered could be tailor-made for the particular person being treated.

Reactions from the chemists

All this seems perfectly reasonable to modern eyes, but in his day Hahnemann was ridiculed and persecuted for his ideas. A rather mercenary motive prompted one stalwart band of critics – the chemists. The doctor's belief in 'micro-doses' – a little achieving a lot – would rapidly put them out of business, they reckoned, and such heresies were not to be tolerated. All over Europe he met with hostility, but in England, his ideas took root. A Frederick Quin set up the hospital in London in 1850 and for some few decades, homeopathy enjoyed considerable interest from the medical profession and the general public.

The rise of allopathy

In the early part of this century, advances made with the other end of the drug-administering spectrum, allopathy (simply speaking, 'bombarding' an illness with a big, powerful counter-drug-dose) put homeopathy in the shade, especially since there are enormous profits to be made in the manufacture of drugs.

Nowadays, renewed attention is being given to the homeopathic school of medicine. A main incentive has been provided by researches into 'mind drugs', for it is well-known that extraordinarily small quantities of these can produce startling effects. Homeopathy, linked with other forms of treatment of mental disorders, may yet have more to offer to patients so far not helped by established medicine and therapy.

A major difficulty lies in the fact that at present homeopathic doctors have to work within orthodox medicine, and take their recruits from people trained in schools where the allopathic method reigns supreme. This runs totally against the whole basis of homeopathy, and means that the discipline is not getting

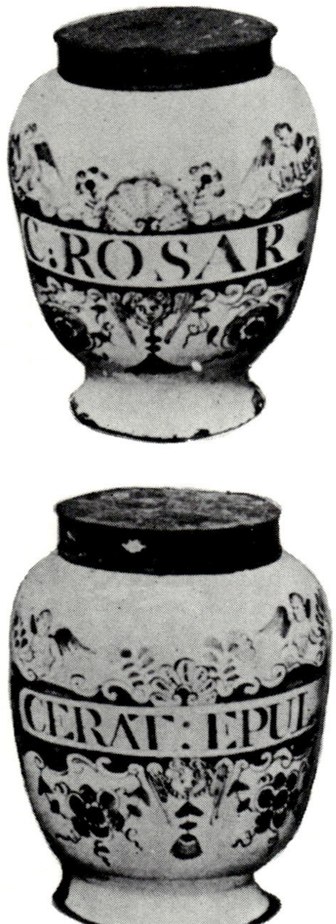

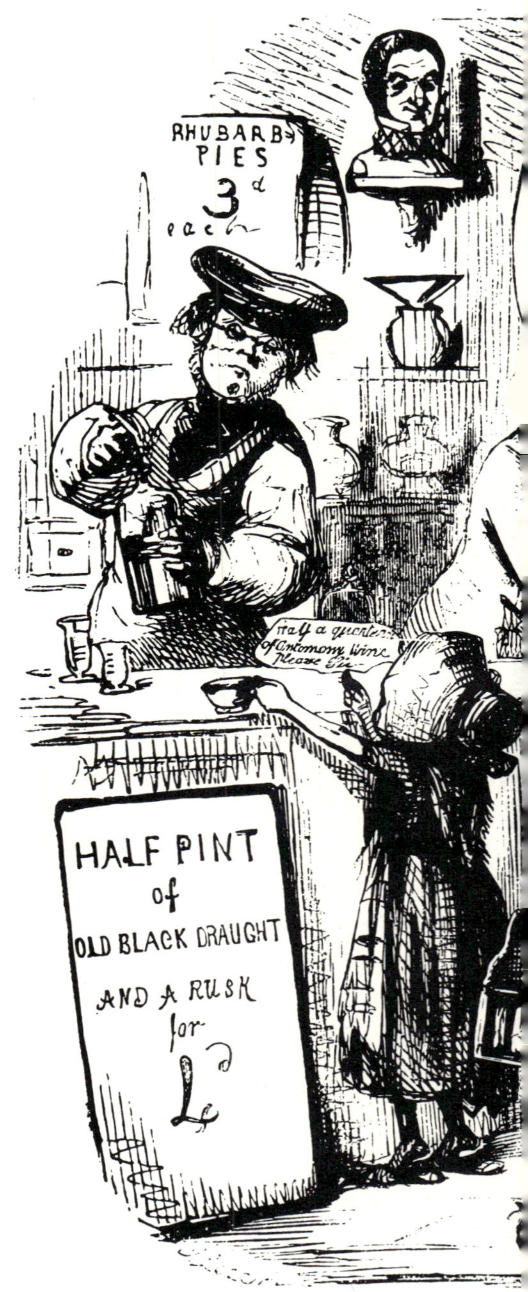

THE MEDICAL MAN,
SIR JAMES

PHYSIC "TO BE

the best brains, the most open and talented minds, to pursue researches further in this field.

World-wide homeopathy

In Britain, homeopathic treatment has always been available under the National Health Service, although in practice it may be difficult to get because there are so few homeopathic doctors. There are six homeopathic hospitals, and ordinary general practitioners can and do take crash courses in homeopathy at the Royal London Homeopathic hospital, and use homeopathic remedies along with the standard drugs. Interest is thought to be slowly increasing, despite some opposition from the medical establishment. In the rest of Europe, homeopathy is widely practised, particularly in Germany and France, where it is very popular.

Russia, with its system of polyclinics, has special homeopathic polyclinics, notably in Moscow and Leningrad. Homeopathy is officially recognized as a speciality in Brazil and India.

In the United States there has been much more opposition to homeopathy, both from the medical establishment and from the powerful drug companies. There are homeopathic hospitals active in San Francisco and also in Pensylvania but no teaching hospital, and a small number of homeopathic practitioners, who have studied in England. Also the American Institute of Homeopathy is active in research. Homeopathy lurks in the half-light of 'fringe medicine', when its theories and contributions could make it a viable alternative to what we know as 'proper' medicine today.

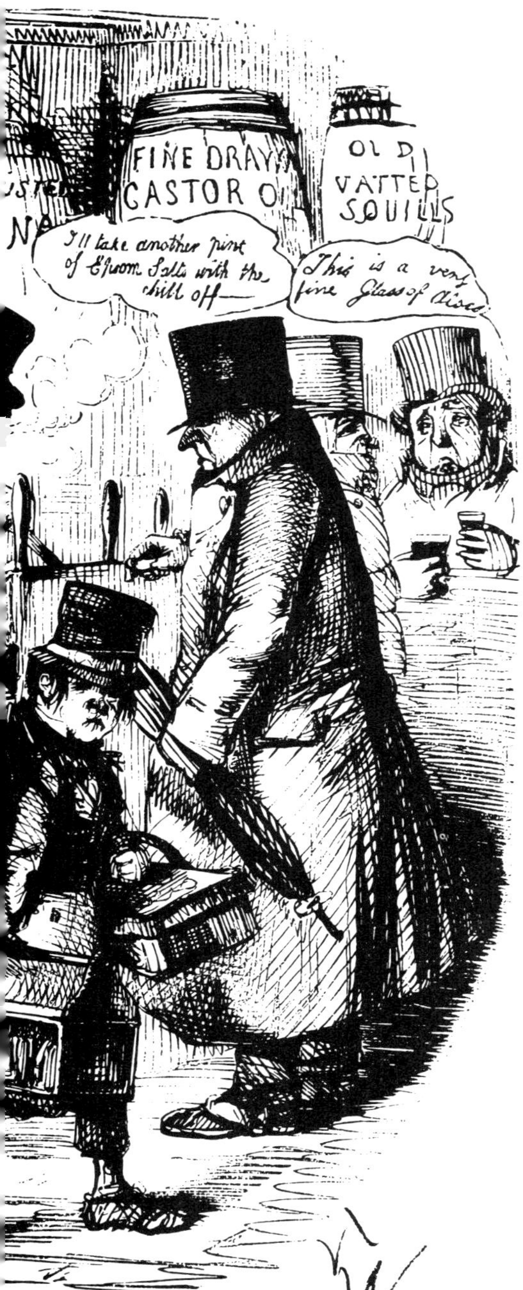
FINE DRAY
CASTOR O
OLD
VATTED
SQUILLS
I'll take another pint of Epsom Salts with the chill off—
This is a very fine Glass of

HE WILL BE, UNDER
AM'S BILL.
THE PREMISES."

Osteopathy

Osteopathy has successfully provided an alternative form of treatment for physical ailments for well over 300 years. Its origins lie in that familiar country figure, the 'bonesetter', and it has never aroused the kind of anger that homeopathy caused because it does not present anything like a threat or a challenge to the mainstream of medical professionals. Manipulation of the bones or joints, either after persistant misuse (say due to bad posture) or after a fracture or dislocation makes the limb stronger and more hardy, but few osteopaths can explain how the 'manipulation' works.

Sometimes, osteopaths go further with claims that handling the body can produce cures for disorders such as epilepsy, tuberculosis, persistent headaches, tumours, and so on. It is possible that massage stimulating the blood system could have a beneficial value for some physical conditions. This is especially the case where the illness has its origin in a disorder of the spinal column, such as spinal lesions, which are common.

Chiropractic

Linked to osteopathy is chiropractic, first developed in the United States by Daniel David Palmer in the mid-nineteenth century. He heard someone complaining that he had lost his hearing years before when he bent over and

Centre *The suspicion that medical men would be tempted to make a business out of dispensing their own drugs is aptly illustrated in this cartoon. The monopoly on drugs is now in the hands of huge companies, and has always been a lucrative business.* **Below** *Although this cartoon of the bonesetter is mocking, in fact many people gain great relief from both osteopathy and chiropractic.*

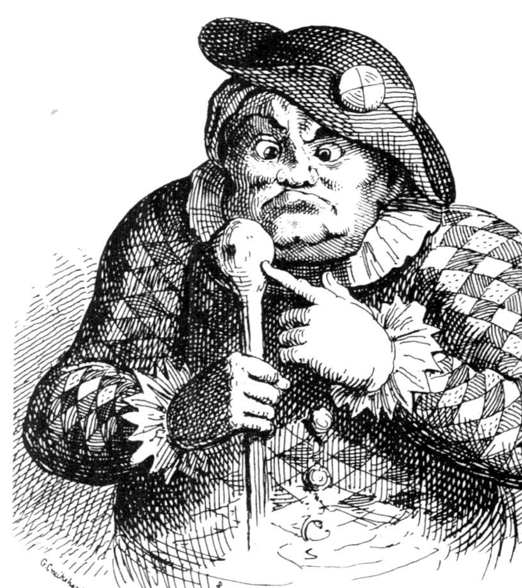

Centre *Buddhist monks reflect the utter serenity of their mental discipline. Eastern systems such as meditation and yoga aim for the perfect combination of spiritual and physical harmony, which results in the balanced individual.*
Extreme right *Western treatment for mental disorders still relies heavily on the theories of Sigmund Freud, pictured here seated among his colleagues.*

something 'went' in his back. Palmer discovered a misplaced vertebra in the man's back and by careful manipulation locked it back into place. Needless to say the man recovered his hearing shortly afterwards.

The basis for chiropractic is an understanding of the main nerve centre, the spinal cord. Even minor derangements, bad posture, or inflammation can cause defective working of the nerves passing up the hollow centre of the cord, with widely disparate results such as the deafness described by Palmer's first case. Chiropractic travelled to Great Britain in the 1900's, and along with osteopathy has achieved wide respectability over recent decades. But chiropractic in America has achieved a much more marked success, with at least 25,000 practitioners by 1960.

Fringe medicine and mental disorders

The various alternative methods of treatment for physical conditions seem comparatively harmless when compared to the considerable upsurge in 'fringe' activities associated with mental disorders. To many people, this represents a dangerous new turn in the long history of unorthodox medicine.

The power of suggestion and the need for faith or confidence are absolute prerequisites in successful curing – but what happens if the mind itself is diseased, and prey to all manner of theories, some ludicrous, some genuinely therapeutic, without the power to distinguish between the two? The complexities of modern life put greater stress on mental equilibrium than ever before, and the increasing use of drugs (legally and illegally) that have a decided effect on the working of the intellect and the shape of the personality add yet more significance to the various activities that have sprung up to help people achieve 'inner peace and harmony'.

Yoga

Yoga is perhaps one of the healthiest and least offensive of the alternative systems currently enjoying high popularity – although fanatics will object to the present interest by pointing out that it is a system of health dating back many thousands of years, to the respiratory therapy system of the Indian and Chinese Buddhists, in the first century AD or even earlier.

The aim of yoga is to enable any man to lift the general standard of his bodily health, and so to improve his mental faculties, and increase his resistance to disease – many of which, as we have seen, owe their origins to psychosomatic imbalances. There are eight steps on the path to improvement: abstention, observance, posture, breath control, sense withdrawal, concentration, meditation and contemplation.

Emphasis is laid on awareness of the spine, and ability to relax the back (which is a reminder of the osteopath's and chiropractic's centre of interest too), while a steadily developed control of breathing is supposed to lead to a greater mental calm and self-control. As with other importations from the east, it is regrettable that only the outward, exercising features of yoga have caught people's attention, and the more serious curative possibilities are hardly explored. Devotees claim for instance that minor troubles such as colds and headaches could be easily self-cured, and immunity to more serious diseases can be built up. Yoga is too readily bound up with romantic

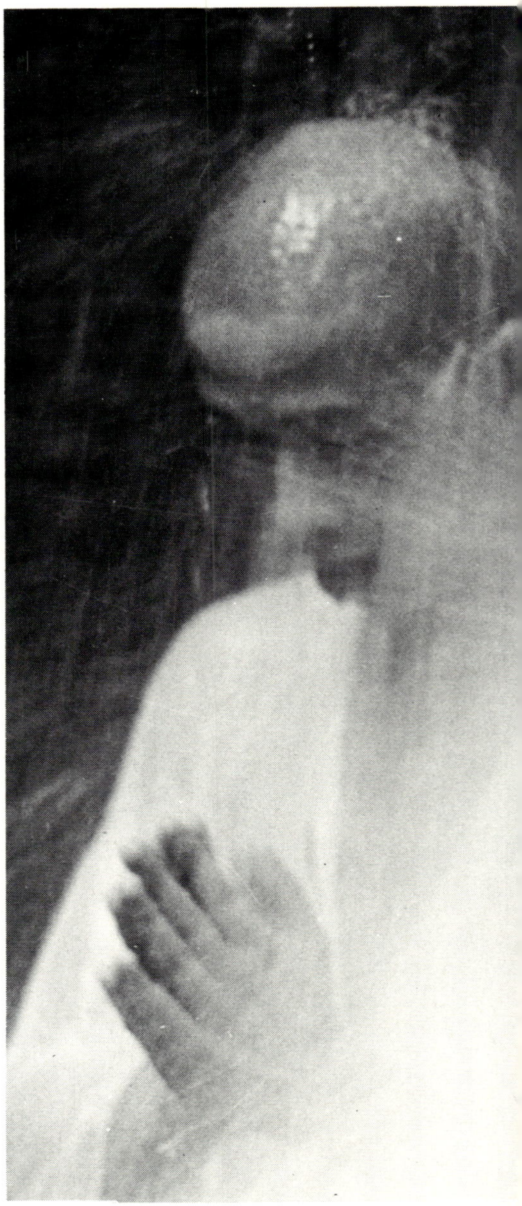

notions of tranquillity and 'transcendental meditation', which is a great pity, for its true value has hardly yet been appreciated in the west.

Medicine and the mind

There are numerous other developments in the treatment of the mind which range from the well-established Freudian psycho-analysis, to psycho-therapy, hypno-therapy, group therapy, and so on, too many to be included in this brief summary. Even more diverse are the workings of spiritual and faith healers, who fall into quite a different category. The aim of any therapist is to help the patient cure *himself*; this imposes a restraint and sense of responsibility on his dealings with the person in his care.

Faith healing and its abuse

The same cannot always be said of the 'healers', many of whom operate on the same basis as quack doctors, evoking a reliance and an emotional response which is thoroughly irresponsible. Faith healing is the subject of intense argument: doctors will say that the illness 'cured' was in the first place wrongly diagnosed, and could have responded to proper treatment. Psychologists will say that the condition may have been psycho-somatic, and the cure the work of auto-suggestion – in other words that the sufferer cured himself, rather than the healer.

In defense of faith healing, it can be said that whatever the explanations, there are thousands of cases where all other remedies have proved useless, and the faith healer at least achieved *results* – which is after all what counts. Just as folk medicine tended to be confined to areas where a measure of success was assured, so it works with faith healing: aches and

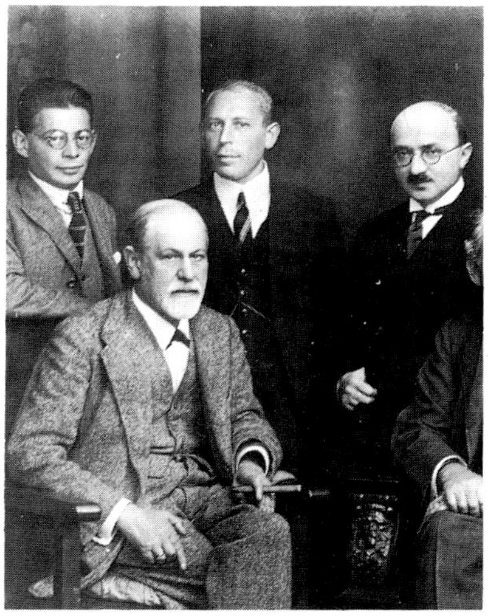

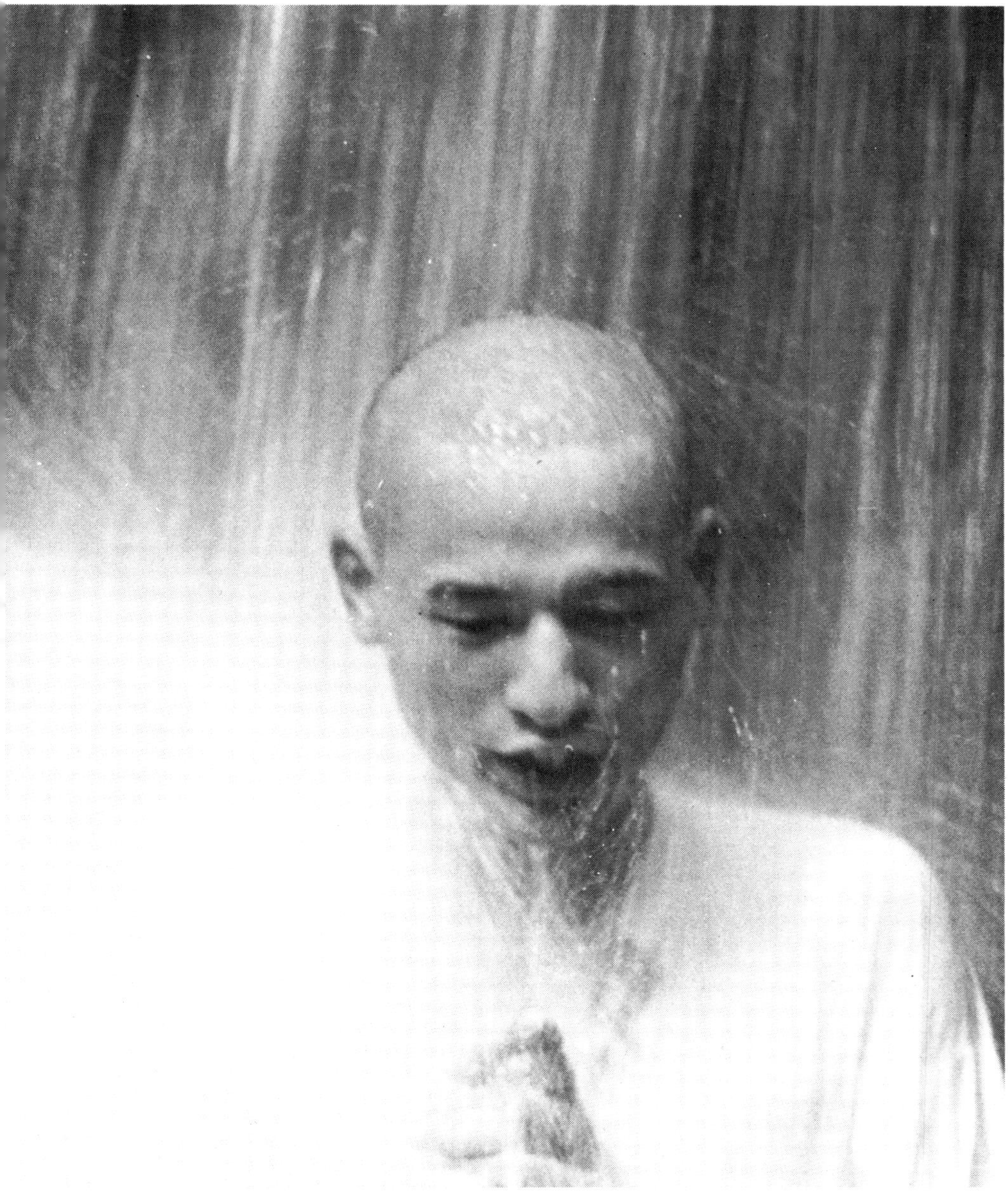

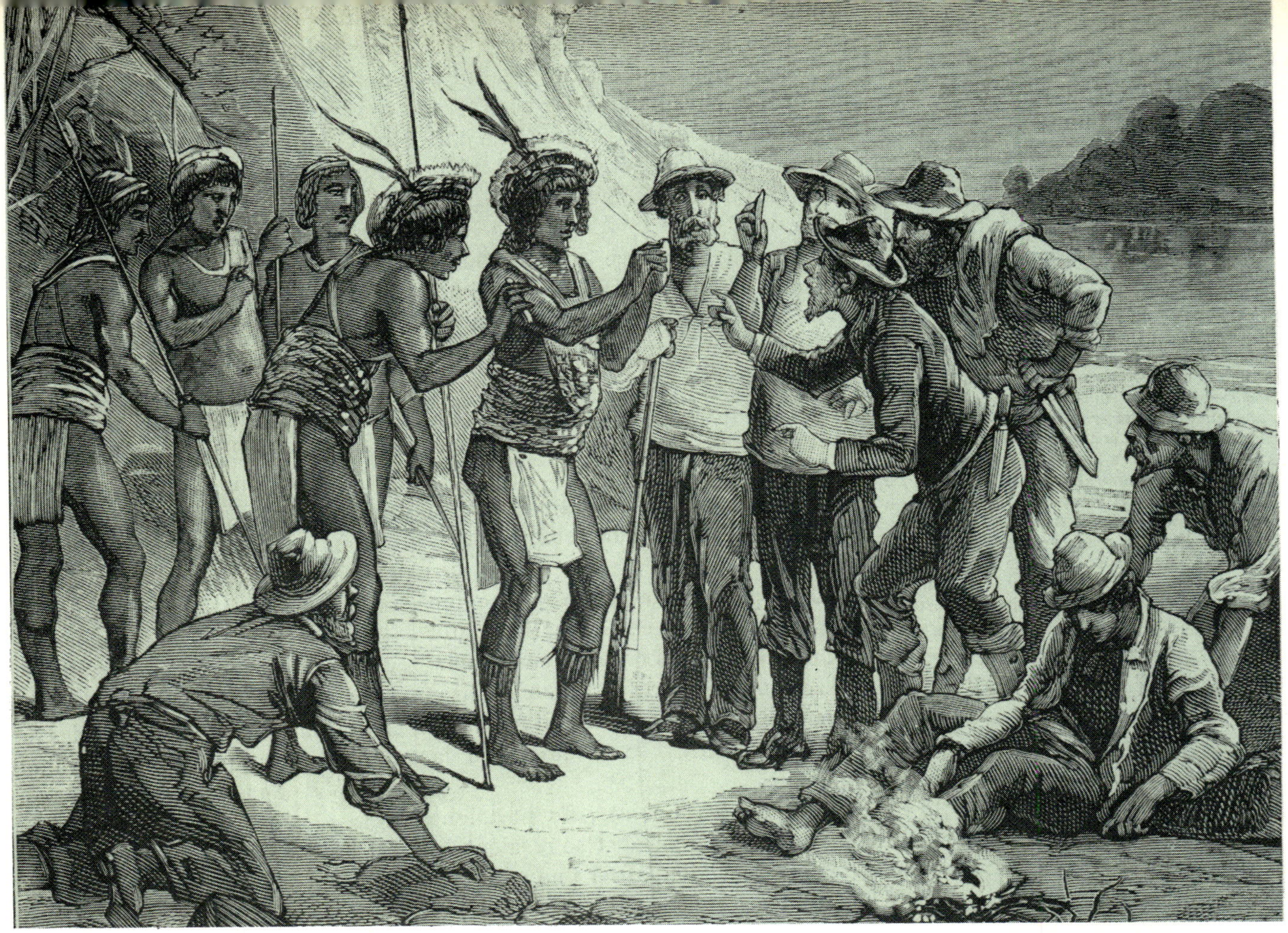

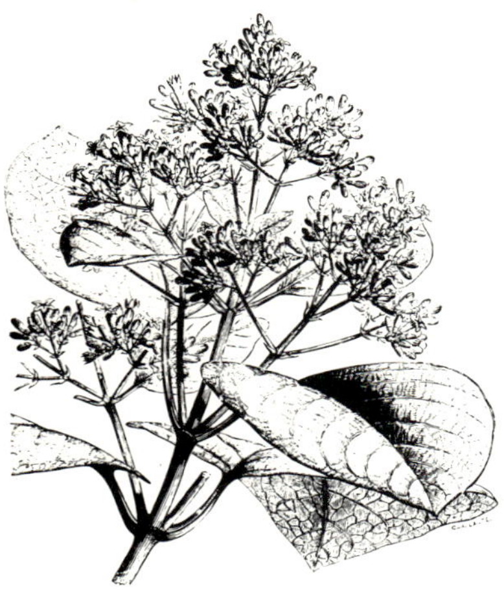

Top *One of the most important medicinal plants* cinchona, *commonly known as quinine, was used by the Peruvian Indians for fevers. Hahnemann based a great deal of his research on this drug. In this nineteenth century engraving, the Indians are showing the bark to white explorers.* **Above** *A detail of the stem and flowers of the plant.*

pains can be made to vanish, skin rashes to heal up, boils to dry, but seldom (if ever) do withered limbs become whole.

Faith healing and cancer

It is sad that one of the greatest areas for faith healing should be in the treatment of cancer. The difficulty is that the term cancer applies to a wide category of illnesses, the true workings of which are still the subject of immensely expensive research. A recent survey in the USA has found no less than 62 specific 'cures', all useless, using diets which include a range of ingredients such as carrot juice with milk; iodine, sulphuric acid, and powdered asbestos. Some cancers do seem to kill themselves off – which leads to speculation about the success of so-called faith healers in this area.

The simple truth was summarized by the American Cancer Society: of every six people who get cancer, two will be saved and four will die. The first two will respond to established treatments. The third will die needlessly, in the sense that he could have been saved if he had received the proper treatment in time. The other three people will die of cancers which cannot be controlled – hence the still present need for medical research, and the folly of believing in any miracle cure for this disease.

A new look at folk medicine

Interestingly, the wheel is coming full circle, linking up folk medicine, with its remedies dating back to the origins of civilization, to the modern quest for new drugs to fight the present incurables like cancer, and the even more experimental areas of mental illnesses like schizophrenia. Botanical drugs – those long used by natives all over the world – are receiving renewed attention from pharmacologists as possible sources of new drug treatments. A leading American scientist, Richard Schultes has said, 'The most important methods for discovering new botanical drugs are the examination of ancient writings; the scientific interpretation of folklore; and field work among primitive peoples still living in close association with the plant world.'

Traditional drugs

There are several world-famous precedents for this approach to medical research. The *cinchona* plant was traditionally used by Peruvian Indians as a cure for fevers; it was first brought to the West by Jesuit priests in 1739. From it, quinine was isolated, the best-known cure for malaria. A synthetic version was created in the 1940's, when World War II cut off supplies from the main production area of the East Indies where it had been smuggled and introduced by the Dutch in the 1800's. To this day, however, the natural product is considered superior to all substitutes. Strains of malaria can build up a resistance to the synthetics, but not to the genuine drug.

From Britain a true folk cure is found in *digitalis*, powdered leaf of the foxglove plant, which is used for heart conditions. It stimulates the vagus centre, monitors the heart beat and has a toning effect on the heart muscle. Its discovery is a quaint story: a Dr William Withering fell in love with a flower painter, Helena Cookes, and because of her took up the habit of plant collecting. In 1775 he heard of a local Shropshire cure for tubercolosis – the foxglove. Intrigued, he began analyzing it, and testing it on himself. In 1785, his famous work 'An Account of the Foxglove' was published, establishing a remedy that still finds acceptance to this day.

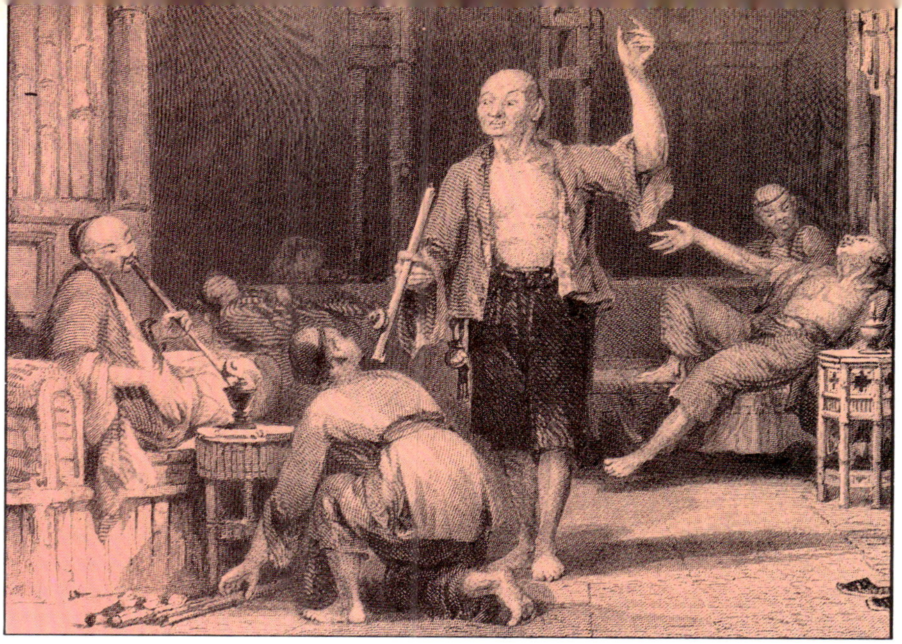

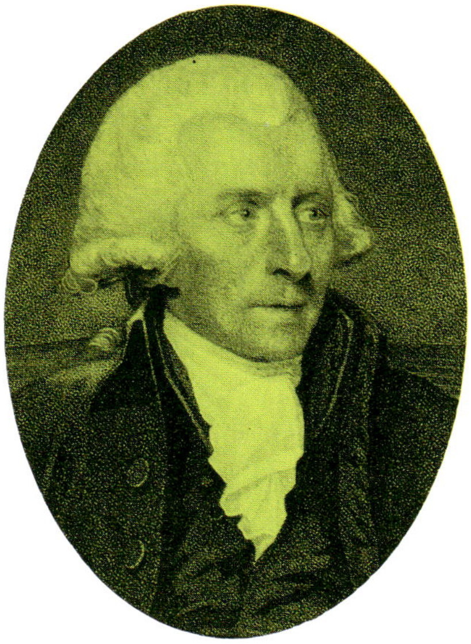

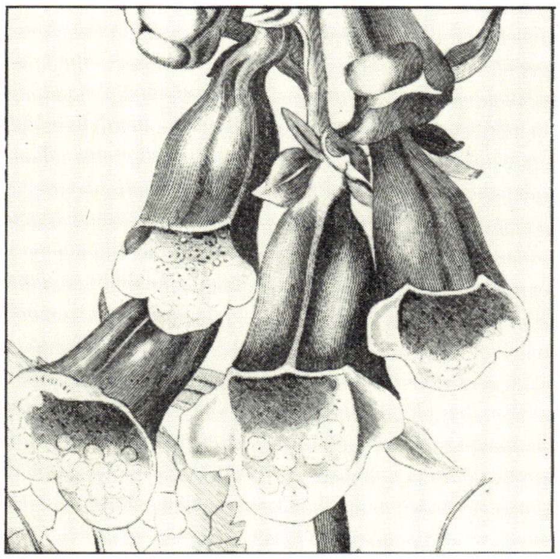

Remedies from the East

The East has yielded several valuable substances, such as *aconite*, used for poisoning arrows by hill tribes in India and China. It was known to the ancient Romans and Greeks: Medea used it for one of her fatal brews. A Viennese doctor, Storck, made the first scientific investigation of it in 1762, since when it has remained recognized officially for the treatment of high blood pressure, or for over-active hearts. (The British Pharmaceutical Code now recommends only the dried root of *Aconitum napellus L.* for use in liniments in the treatment of sciatica and rheumatism. It induces a tingling, followed by numbness, and has a mildly stimulating effect.)

Another eastern drug recommended originally in ancient Chinese and Indian writings, is *chaulmoogra* from the rare tree *Hydnocarpis wightiana* growing in remote spots of India, Burma and Malaya. This was a folk remedy introduced to the west by a doctor in the

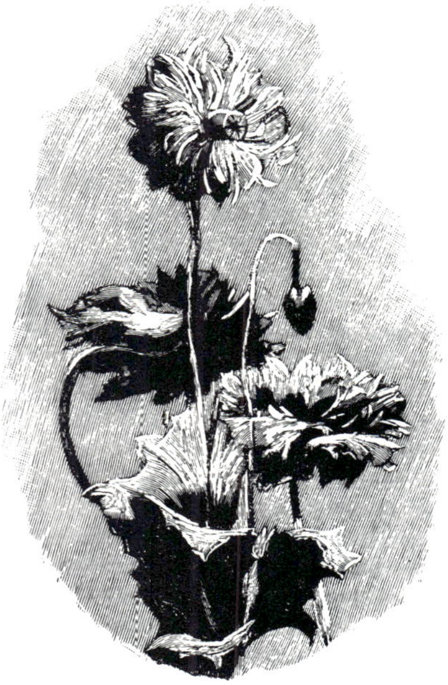

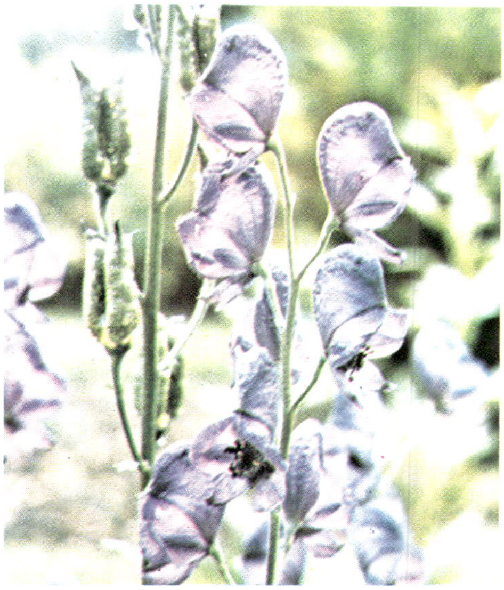

Top *Opium was used in China as a sedative and relaxant.* **Above** *A detail of the opium flower and leaves.* **Above left** *Dr* William *Withering who discovered the medicinal properties of the foxglove.* **Below left** *A detail of the foxglove, from which the drug* digitalis *is made to treat heart conditions.* **Left** *Aconite has a long history of use as a poison. It is now used to treat rheumatism in liniments, and is also a homeopathic remedy for colds and fevers.*

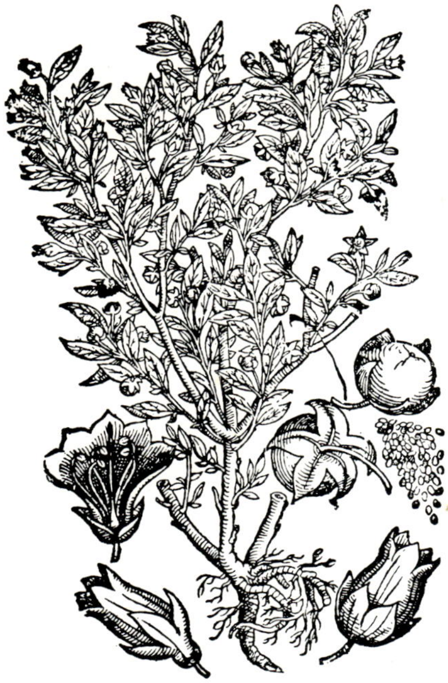

Indian Medical Service; oil expressed from the seeds is useful for the treatment of leprosy and other skin diseases.

Belladonna was also known to the ancient Indians, although we tend to associate it with limpid-eyed ladies of Renaissance Italy, who adopted it as a way of dilating their pupils and making their eyes large and shining. It has many medical uses, as it contains *atropine* with an anaesthetic effect. Small doses have been tried for excessive peristalsis and colic pains; gastric and duodenal ulcers respond with its application. It was once used for eye surgery, to dilate the pupil, but nowadays *homatropine* is preferred as the effects of *atropine* are prolonged.

Narcotics from folk medicine

The greatest challenge for the experimental pharmacologist lies with the field of narcotic drugs – these too have a long history in folk medicine, and it is hoped they will continue to yield valuable substances in particular for the treatment of mental illness. One of the most striking finds in this area was *rauwolfia*. Present-day Nigerian witch-doctors use the roots boiled up in a decoction to help patients 'possessed' by some evil spirit.

It has also figured in Indian Sanskrit writings dating back 3,000 years BC, where it is called *sarpagandha*, a treatment for snakebites and lunacy. Serious study of the plant in the west began in the 1930's but it was not until the 1950's that a drug emerged from the laboratories: *Rauwolfia serpentina* had yielded up *Raudixin*. By 1957 it was in wide use for cases of schizophrenia, paranoia, manic states, chronic alcoholism and withdrawal symptoms in narcotic addiction.

A new alkaloid produced in 1952, *reserpine* was synthesized (manufactured chemically) in 1956 and has taken over from the natural substance. Two other narcotic drugs, *coca* and *peyote* from

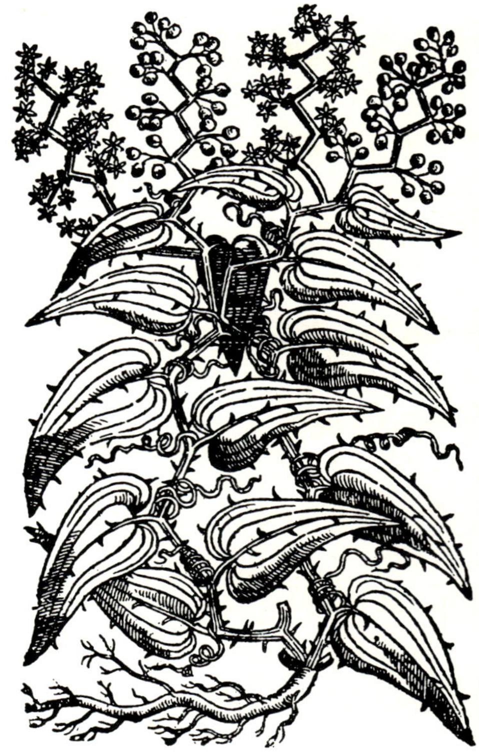

South America are painkillers long used by the Indians; the first yields cocaine, widely used in dentistry.

Numerous members of the *Datura* family are known to natives in southern USA, Mexico, and South America. The Incas used a tree variety, *datura fastuosa*, to numb people before ritual surgery or sacrifice. An American *datura*, 'Jimson Weed' popular for Red Indian peace pipes and as a relaxant, has proved useful (in small doses) for the relief of asthma. This too contains *atropine*, like belladonna, with an anaesthetic effect.

More research needs to be done on LSD, derived from the fungus *ergot Claviceps purpurea*. The ancient Assyrians used it as a medicine, and for hundreds of years it has cropped up in folk cures to relieve haemorrhaging, usually post-

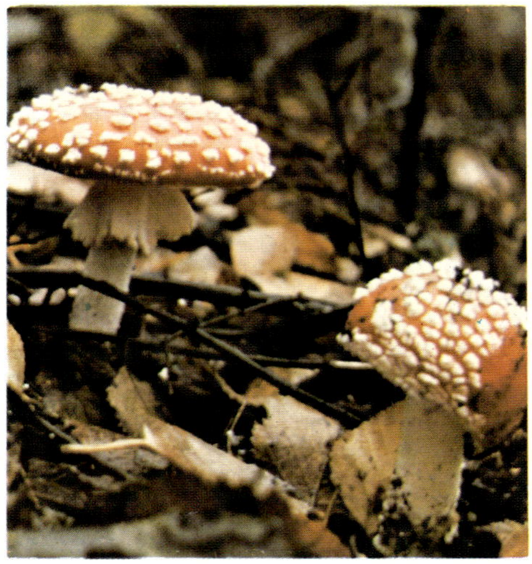

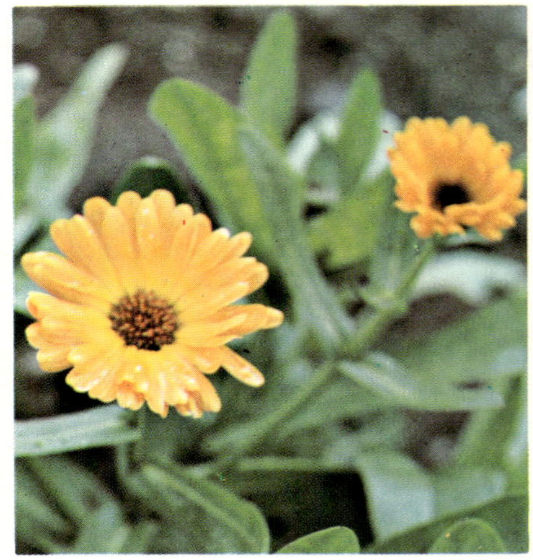

Above right *Sarsparilla was originally used by the American Indians for cough remedies. Analysis shows that the root has stimulant and sweat-inducing properties.* **Above left** *Belladonna or Deadly nightshade contains* atropin. **Below right** *Marigold is used in ointment as a homeopathic treatment for cuts.* **Below left** *The toadstool Fly Agaric is yet another homeopathic remedy, used to treat nervous disorders.*

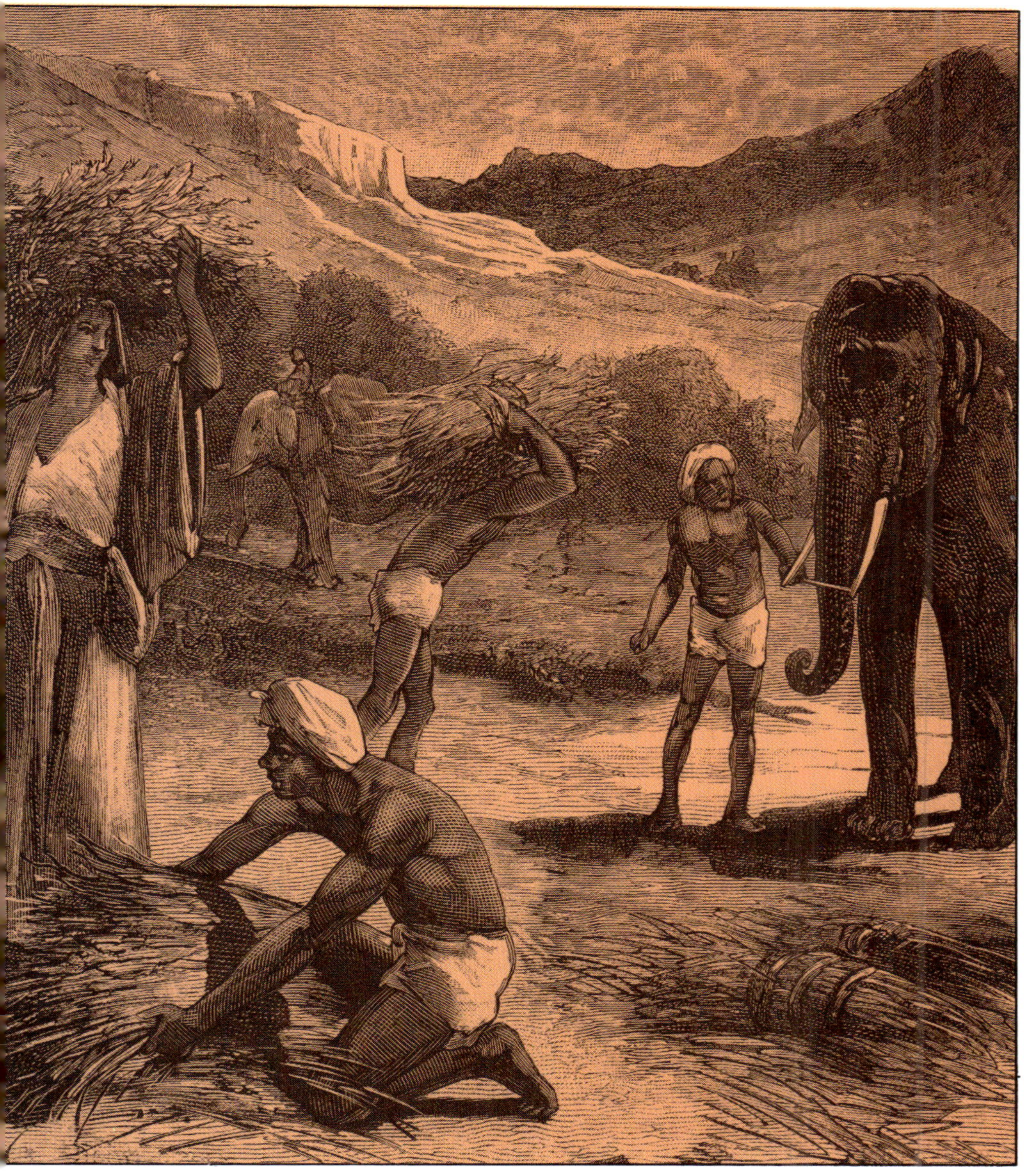

Above left *A nineteenth century engraving showing the harvest of sarsparilla in India.* **Below left** *The American Indian medicine man knew the healing properties of many plants and herbs which are only now being rediscovered.* **Below centre** *Ergot derivatives are made from the fungus on the bark of willow trees, a detail of a willow is shown here.* **Below right** *A delightful nineteenth century engraving of a botanist closely examining a specimen under his glass.*

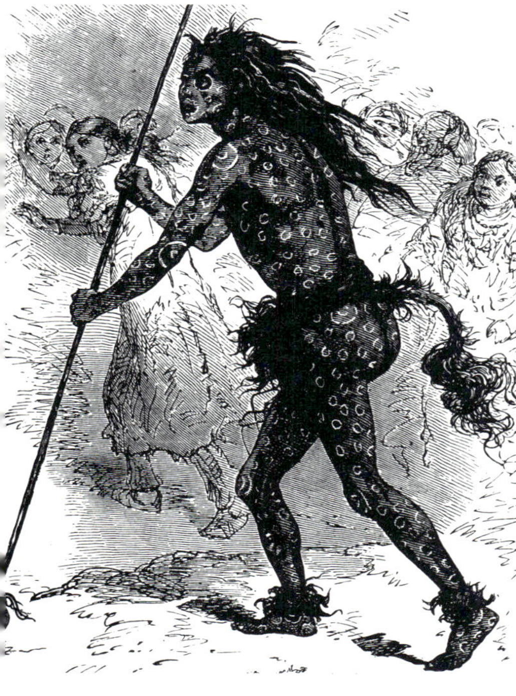

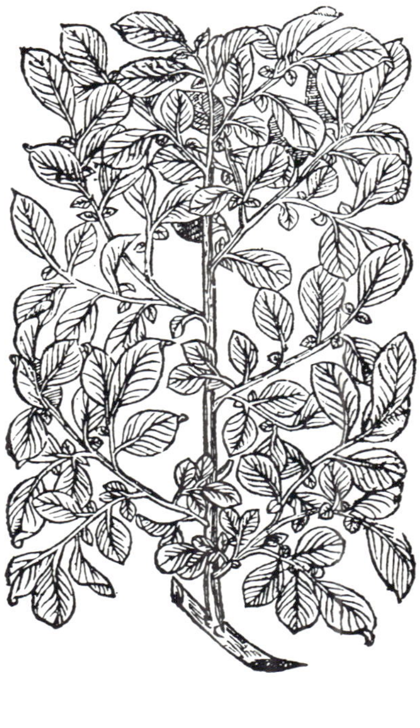

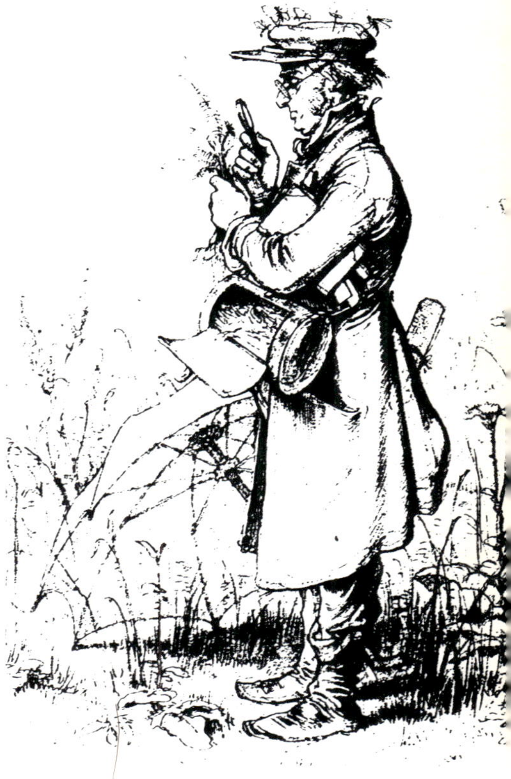

partum. An ergot alkaloid, *ergometrine* is now used as a uterine stimulant, while another, *ergotamine* has proved useful for migraine. But further work is held up because of the problems of drug addiction, black marketeering, and illegality that surround its importation and study in the USA.

Potential for the future

These are just a few of the significant finds from the world of folk medicine. There are many more to come: American Indians have long used Yucca leaves and edible yams as a remedy, and now we know they contain saponins, useful in the development of hormonal treatments. Seaweed was used by the ancient Chinese for dropsy, abscesses, and certain forms of skin cancer. South Sea Islanders and Latin American Indians have the same traditions. Western medicine's knowledge of the beneficial properties of seaweeds, mosses, and lichens is still in its infancy.

It would be a foolish error to attribute more than is just to the herb-women, priests, hermits and farmers who universally have been the originators of folk remedies. Most of their discoveries were haphazard, not scientific – and history does not record the sad stories of herbalists who died choking on some luscious but lethal berry, or who were murdered by enraged relatives after an unfortunate prescription had gone wrong. But modern scientific medicine can learn two immensely important qualities from the long and intriguing history of folk medicine: first, a greater respect for the wonders of nature, and less pride in the concoctions of the chemist's shelf; secondly, a greater awareness of the psychological aspect of all illnesses, both in their origins and in their treatment.

A happy, secure patient is sure to get well. A nervous man, blinded with incomprehensible jargon, will find little relief. Western medicine has immeasurably improved conditions in such areas as surgery, childbirth, dangerous diseases of infancy, and so on, but for the vast array of average upsets and disorders, it still has failures.

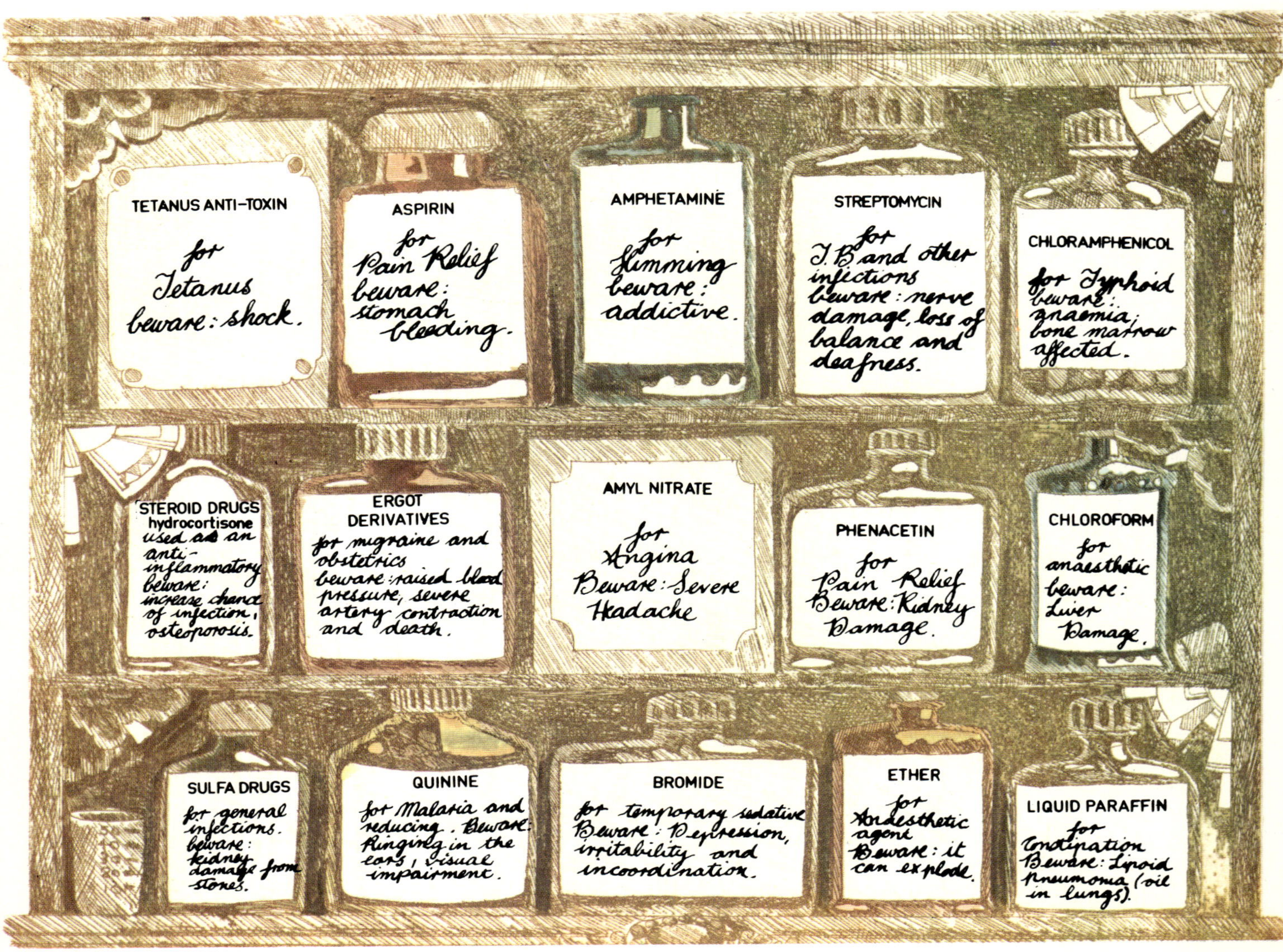

Below *A sketch of a medical cupboard showing a wide range of drugs, along with their sources and side-effects in treatment.*

Folk Medicine Remedies and Cures

In the following pages you will find folk remedies from all over the world. Many of the ingredients are still used in medicine today, while others are weird and wonderful flights of the imagination. Though some are both harmless and effective, like using dock leaves to soothe nettle stings, you should be very wary of using these cures, because some plants can have dangerous side effects. Anyone interested would be wise not to try them, but should investigate the stock of the nearest herbal or homeopathic supplier.

Stomach disorders

The ancient Peruvians used the pulverized seeds of a woody vine, *Mucuna elliptica* as a purgative. (Confirmed usage by modern doctors.)

Traditional Peruvian

The yellow bark of the barberry *Berberis vulgaris* in ale or white wine, makes an excellent purgative drink, and a good tonic.

Traditional English

Diuretics

A decoction of the roots and seed of parsley is a well-known cleanser of the system, and acts as a diuretic. So also does dandelion tea, known in many country areas as piss-in-bed. In France it goes also by the name *piss-en-lit*.

Traditional English

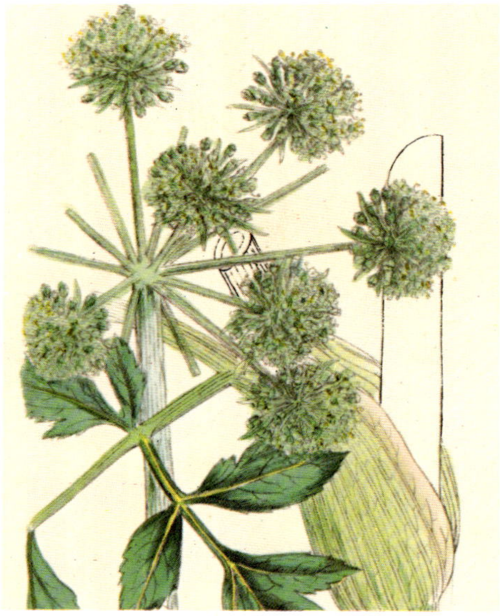

Angelica aids digestion.

The two varieties of the Manuka tree (L.scoparium) are extremely valuable in Maori folk medicine. Pieces of the bark were boiled until the water darkened, and the resulting liquid was taken for constipation. The boiled seed capsules produced a fluid which would cure diarrhoea and dysentery. And an infusion of the leaves produced an effective diuretic. These are only a few of the uses of this most valuable little tree.

New Zealand/Maori Folk Medicine

Bed wetting

Take some haws, put them in a vessel of red earthenware, mix therewith a good quantity of honey, then put in an oven with bread; of this take four spoonfuls three times a day, for a diuretic effect.

Traditional Welsh

For bed-wetting, an old English cure used to be a portion of cooked mouse.

Traditional English

Wind

For wind in the stomach: $\frac{1}{2}$ pint of milk and 4 teaspoons of fine soot. This is a folk remedy variant of official treatment for flatulent conditions of the stomach and intestines, when carbon is prescribed, as it absorbs stomach gases.

Traditional Irish

Haemorrhoids

$\frac{1}{2}$lb of carobs (St John's sweetbread, *Seratonia siliqua)* chopped and put in a quart of vodka; keep in a warm place for ten days minimum. Take one tot twice daily, before meals.

Siberian remedy

Piles were treated by the Maoris by boiling the leaves of the Kopakopa (plantain), and either bathing with the hot liquid, or using it as a steam bath to reduce the swelling.

New Zealand/Maori Folk Medicine

Wild buttercup roots boiled with lard to make an ointment is good for piles, or, set fire to a tarred rope, place it in a metal bucket and squat over the fumes. Some find a poultice of boiled onions a relief – even others apply this with oil and vinegar, but the acid of the vinegar would be too sharp.

Traditional Welsh

Take smoked dried goat's flesh, dessicate completely, and reduce to as fine a powder as you can; lay thereof on live coals in a fire-proof utensil, and put the same in a commode and sit thereon.

Traditional Welsh

Oil of turpentine with herb *artemisia* and the *Datura stramonium* (a well-known narcotic plant) are an old remedy ointment for piles.

Mexican Folk Medicine

Camphor and blue copperas is added to fresh pork shin bone marrow, kept cold and applied externally, for piles.

Traditional Chinese

Laxative tonic

Cassia leaves (*C. acutifolia*) three parts
Buckthorn bark (*Frangula alnus*) two parts
Cascara, fruit (*Rhamus catharica*) two parts
Anis, fruit (*Anisum vulgare*) one part
Licorice root (*Glycyrrhiza glarba*) one part
One tablespoon to $1\frac{1}{2}$ cups of boiling water; infuse for 25 to 30 minutes, then strain. Take one-third to half a cup at night before bed.

Russian Folk Medicine

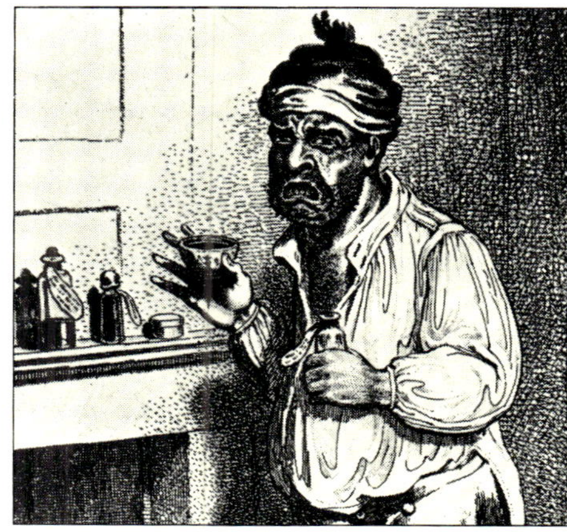

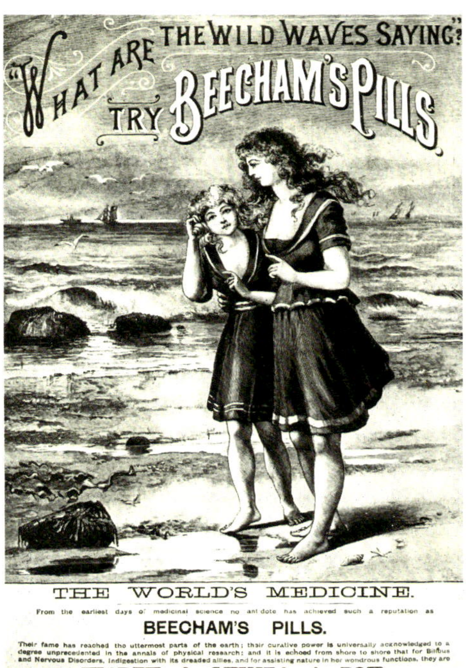

The gum of the thorny bush, a species of Acacia, is used as a laxative.

African Folk Medicine

In various parts of Africa, varieties of the *Ranunculaceae* contain an oily acrid liquid yielding *anemonin*. Examples are the anemone, the virgin's bower (Clematis) or the buttercup. The roots and leaves dried, powdered, and taken act as counter-irritants or purgatives, and are widely used.

African Folk Medicine

Cascara sagrada was long used by the Indians of the Pacific coast as a laxative long before it became so popular with settlers. Spanish priests were among the first white people to adopt the practice.

'There is a kind of parsley called in Welsh *perllys yr hel*, because it grows in such places as are occasionally overflowed by the tide, and is of a salt nature. In Latin it is called *Petroselinum marinum*, and is good in all obstructions of the urine and humors of the body, as well as colic and strangury, the juice being taken. The juice is useful to destroy unhealthy granulations in a wound. It will grow in gardens, where it should be kept wherever the sea is distant'.

Traditional Welsh

Diarrhoea
For diarrhoea, the ancient Aztecs had a remedy still used in folk medicine in Mexico today: pulverized avocado seed is mixed with plantain water – or sometimes powdered charcoal instead, for use as an enema.

Mexican Folk Medicine

An old bush remedy for diarrhoea or dysentery was the bloodwood tree. It exudes a reddish gum, which if swallowed in sufficient quantity was claimed to be most effective – too effective, some folk said.

Traditional Australian

Chop finely 1lb of figs and 2oz senna leaves. Add a cupful of treacle, mix well and put into earthenware pots. Adults may take $\frac{1}{2}$ teaspoonful, children half this dose.

Welsh/English border

Worms
The Cherokee Indians used the pinkroot (*Spigelia marilandica*), powdering the fresh root, as a cure for worms. This remedy was adopted by the white settlers, and only went out of fashion because travelling herbalists diluted the real powder with useless varieties. A member of the *Logania* family, the pinkroot has trumpet-shaped flowers, bright red outside, yellow within, on a single stem.

American Indian

An old cure for worms is to take the hair from a horse's forelock, and eat it on bread and butter.

Traditional English

In Ancient Hindu writings, the pomegranate figures as a cure forworms. In 1805 a scientist called Buchanan discovered *pelletierine tannate* in pomegranate, a useful remedy for the tapeworm.

Indian Folk Medicine

The Papaw tree (*Carica Papaya*) is used by the natives as a cure for worms. The fresh milky juice from the fruit, preferably a little under-ripe, is best.

Indian Folk Medicine

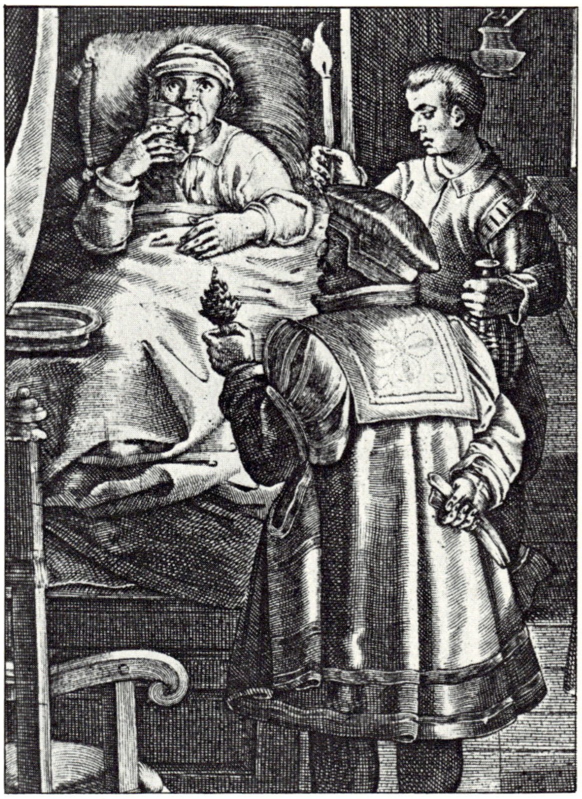

Administering a purgative.

Indigestion
The plantain herb (*Plantago*) has seeds which, if soaked in water, yield a mucilage (a gummy fluid). If the seeds are taken whole, they swell and give off this fluid in the intestines. This makes an excellent digestive aid, and was adopted by the English colonials as a remedy of long standing for stomach disorders.

Indian Folk Medicine

An old Siberian remedy for indigestion is to take plantain seeds in water, when they form a thick mass.

Russian Folk Medicine

FINIS

Jaundice and liver complaints

Jaundice
'The following are the virtues of the nettle. Take the juice of this herb mixed with white wine, strain carefully and let it cool. Drink some thereof night and morning; it will cure you of the jaundice, renovate the blood, and remove any disease existing therein. If the juice is taken, mixed half and half with barley wort, it will cure the pleurisy in the side, and will renovate and invigorate an aged man in body and mind. If the seed of the nettle in powder is taken, mixed with wine, it is very useful for wind colic, strangury, or a chronic cough, and will reduce a swelling, producing a flow of urine without harm to the bladder.'

Traditional Welsh

Thirteen cloves of garlic at the end of a cord, worn around the neck for thirteen days, are considered a safeguard against jaundice – but the wearer must, in the middle of the night of the thirteenth day, go to the corner of two streets, take off his garlic necklet, and flinging it behind him, run home without turning round to see what has become of it.

Old Cuban Remedy

A live spider, rolled up in butter and taken as a pill is a cure for jaundice.

West Sussex remedy

In New England, USA, a live spider is taken in a spoonful of molasses as a cure for jaundice.

New England Folk Medicine

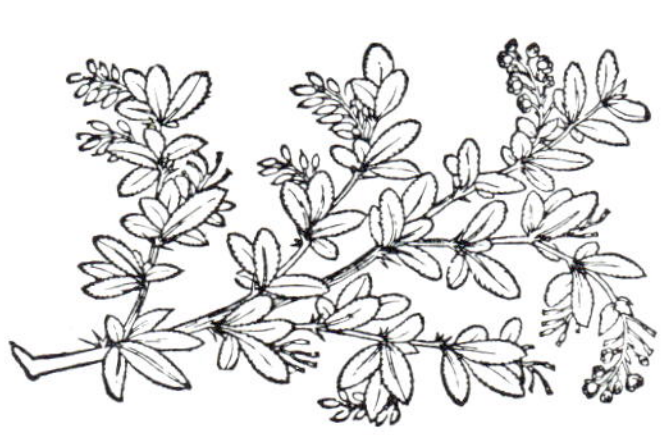

The barberry plant.

Barberry tea (*Berberis vulgaris*) is good for gallstone and jaundice.

Lincolnshire remedy

In Mexico, take medicine with the right hand for liver complaints, and the left for the kidneys.

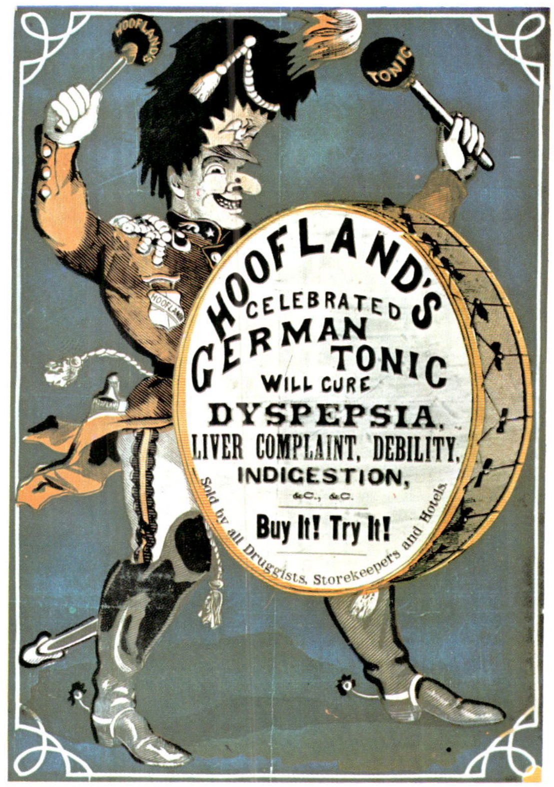

Dandelion liver tonic
4oz fresh roots, boiled in two pints of water until the liquid is reduced to one pint. Strain off and take a wineglassful twice a day. This drink is also good for rheumatism.

Traditional Welsh/English

Fresh dill pickle juice, combined with an equal part of fresh tomato juice is a good summer remedy for liver complaints. Take half a cup, three times daily, after meals.

Southern Russian remedy

FINIS

Coughs, colds and bronchitis

In Flemish folk lore, anyone who has the ague should go early in the morning to an old willow, make three knots in one of its branches, and say "God Morrow, old one; I give thee the cold – good morrow, old one."

Traditional Flemish

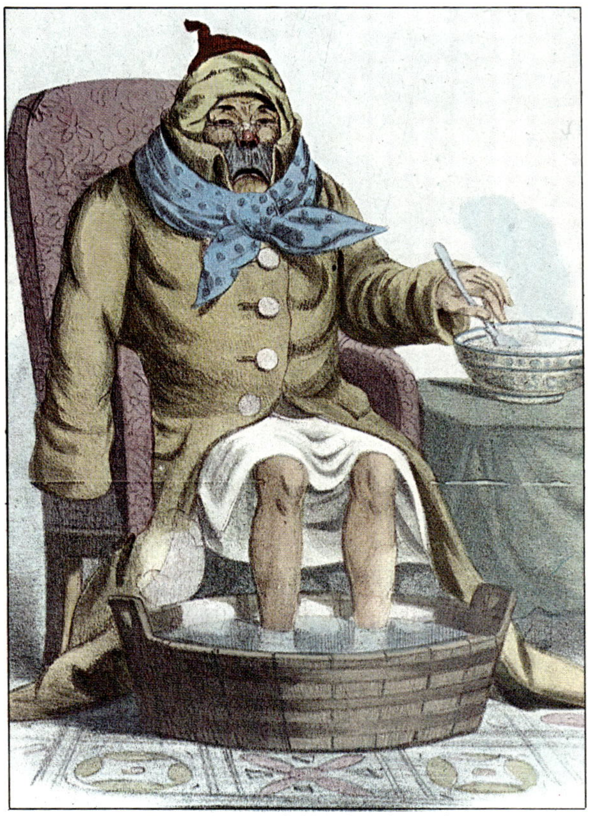

The misery of the common cold.

A German cure for ague is to walk round an oak and say,
'Good evening, thou good one old,
I bring thee the warm and the cold'

In England and Ireland, sickly children are passed through a split oak in order that they gather strength from the tree . . .

Transference Cures

'To make ye horse dunge water, for Agues and feavers and all distempers. Take horse dunge and putt to it so much Ale as will make it like hasty puding, and put it into your still. Then putt on ye topp one pound of treakell, and a quarter of a pound of genger in powder and the same in sweet anisseeds, and so distill all these together. This water also is good for women in labor and in childbed.'

Elizabethan English

A favourite Australian remedy was horehound – picked by the roadside. The plant was boiled and mixed with honey – a great cure for colds, but very unpleasant to taste.

Australian Folk Medicine

For bronchitis, wear a piece of brown paper, pierced with holes, around the neck at night in bed. Another good cure is to wear next to the throat the foot part of the stocking or sock you wore during the previous day.

Australian Folk Medicine

To relieve infant's colds: 1 teaspoon of pure olive oil, 1 teaspoon of honey, the juice of a lemon, added to a stiffly beaten white of 1 egg. Given at short intervals it is remarkably good.

Australian Folk Medicine

For a cough, make a hole through a lemon, and fill it with honey, Roast the lemon, then strain the juice. Take a teaspoon of it frequently. *Or*, cut a hole in the middle of a swede, fill it with brown sugar, and leave it to stand overnight. A juice will collect – take it next day. *Or*, try two or three snails, boiled in barley water.

Welsh/English border

The soft white gum of the Manuka tree was chewed to relieve a severe cough.

New Zealand/Maori Folk Medicine

The balsam poplar (*Populus tacamahaca*) has leaf buds that yield a resinous exudate, with an invigorating balsamic odour. The Pillager Ojibwa

Indians used to make a salve with it by mixing it up with bear or mutton fat, and pressing a small ball up the nostrils to ease bronchitis.

This substance was a recognized drug, listed in the National Formulary from 1916 to 1965. It is used, as are the turpentines, and recognized as an expectorant in 'subacute or chronic bronchitis.' Called the 'tacamahac' tree, it is found along streams and lakesides from NewFoundland to Alaska, and in other parts of North USA.

American Folk Medicine

Elder leaves or elder flower tea is good taken internally for catarrh, colds, and inflammation.

Traditional English

A cure for the common cold: egg white, honey, linseed oil, sugar and mulled stout are all good. Hot milk and rum are also recommended. For a tickling cough a Dublin mixture is to take equal parts of porter and milk, sweetened with sugar to taste. Or try a small pat of butter rolled in sugar.

Traditional Irish

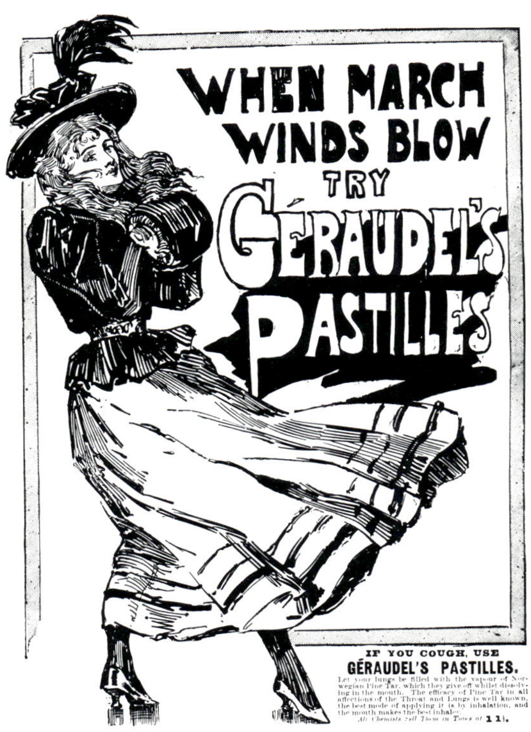

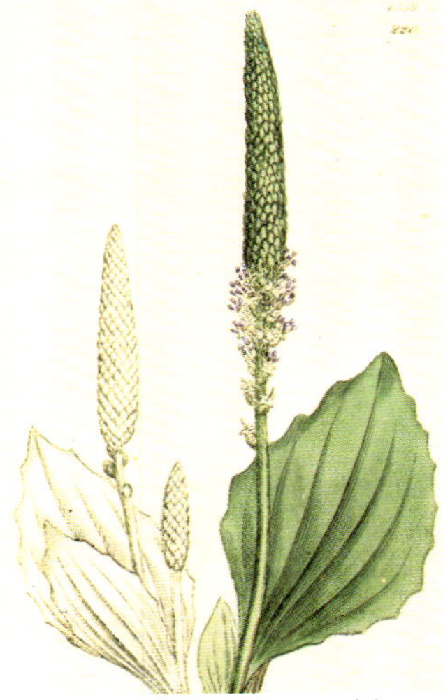

Plantain helps cure colds.

A traditional method that still holds good is to steep willow leaves in hot water, and drink the resulting tea. The leaves contain acetyl-salicylic acid, with an effect like aspirin. Traditionally the rest of the liquid is poured over the head, which would also have the correct effect of helping to lower the body temperature.

Mexican remedy

In New Zealand the attractive shrub called Rumarahan (*Pomaderns kumeraho*) has excellent curative properties for colds, asthma, bronchitis and chest complaints. The liquid resulting from steeping the leaves in water was taken internally for colds, asthma and bronchitis. It is also a well-known herbal cure in ointment form for skin diseases.

New Zealand/Maori Folk Medicine

A good remedy to try is onions boiled in molasses. Take the resulting syrup.

Welsh/English border

An Irish recipe for sore throat is a cabbage leaf tied round the throat, and the juice of the cabbage taken with honey used to be given for hoarseness.

Traditional Irish

The Maoris of New Zealand used the nectar from the crimson flowers of the Rata tree.

New Zealand/Maori Folk Medicine

A Saint's Day cure for a sore throat is St Brigid's Cotton: a piece of cloth left outside the door of the house on the night before February 1. On the feast of St. Brigid, she passes and blesses the cloth. The sufferer keeps the cloth and ties it round his throat whenever he has this ailment.

Traditional Irish

In New England, the skin of a black cat is considered a good remedy for sore throat, tied round the neck.

American Folk Medicine

Boil equal parts of sage, rosemary, honeysuckle and plantain in water. Be sure the water covers the leaves. Add a tablespoon of honey to each pint of liquid. The resulting infusion makes a good hairwash, and a good gargle for sore throat or sore mouth.

Welsh/English border

Licorice boiled in water is good for coughs, or problems of the breast and lungs.

Traditional English

Old Siberians would wear red flannel wristlets to help keep off colds and chills, or put a potato amulet in their pockets as a preventive measure. Another method was to put dry mustard inside their socks before going out to work. Other cures were rubbing the chest with pork fat, or a rub-down with poppy seed oil – this last remedy coming from old Amur Province in Far East Russia.

Russian Folk Medicine

Croup

A cold water compress consisting of a man's handkerchief, well wrung out, was placed around the throat and covered with a warm scarf. As an extra, onions were chopped up and put in a pillowcase and the feet of the patient were placed in this and left for as long as necessary.

Australian Folk Medicine

Whooping cough

This used to be a very serious condition in small babies, under a year old, and caused the death of many. It is therefore not surprising that folk remedies should abound for this condition, which consists of spasms of coughing so severe that the infant appears to choke, ending with a whooping noise. Vomiting often occurs during the attacks. It can be a long drawn out illness. Nowadays it is hardly ever so serious.

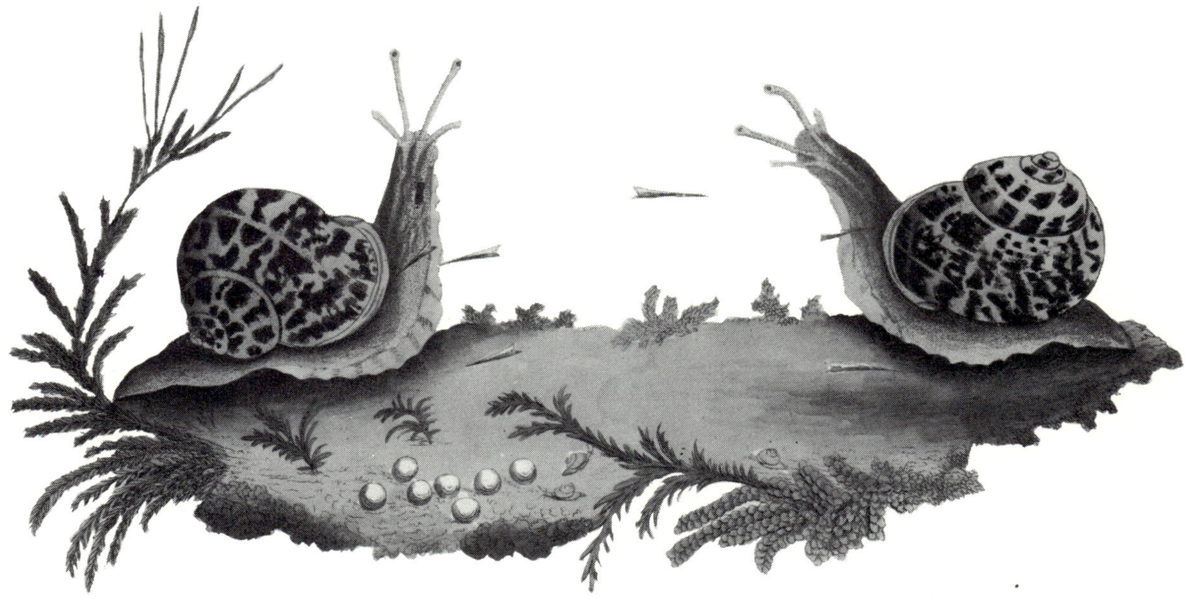

A gypsy cure was to let a snail crawl over brown sugar, and when the sugar was soaked in the slime, it was given to the patient to eat.

Traditional English

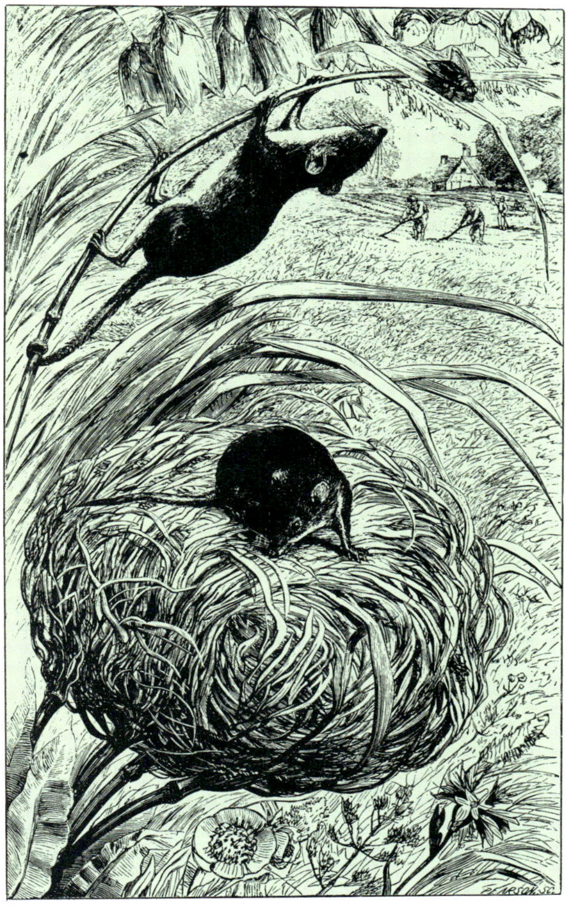

Take a large whitestone turnip raw, and cut it in slices as thin as possible. Lay these on a large plate and sprinkle them freely with sugar, allowing to stand until the juice flows freely, and the sugar dissolves. For a baby, give one small teaspoon every few hours until relieved; for older ones, a larger dose in proportion.

Australian Folk Medicine

The first and last piece of the breakfast of a husband and wife of the same surnames before marriage is given to the child. On old days in County Clare and County Longford, the parents were to go out looking for a man on a white horse and ask him "Man of the white horse, what is the cure for this disease?" and do whatever the man said in answer.

Traditional Irish

A child was passed over a bramble bush seven times, with the following words: 'In bramble, out cough,
Here I leave the whooping cough'

Essex transference cure

In the West Indies, a strip of red cloth is worn round the neck as a preventive measure for small children.

West Indian Folk Medicine

In Gloucestershire, roasted mouse was considered a good remedy for whooping cough. The same is found all over the world.

Traditional English

Asthma

For asthma, it used to be considered helpful to swallow a handful of spider's webs rolled into a ball. This is common to English, European, and Australian folk medicine. In 1882 it was discovered that spider's webs contain *arachnidin*, a powerful febrifuge, that would help to bring down high temperatures.

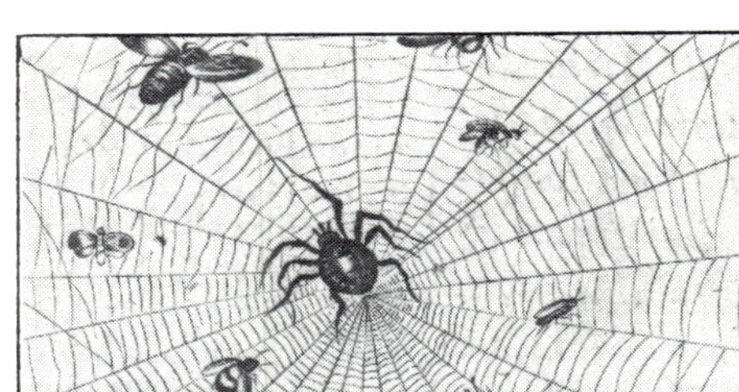

To relieve asthma, make a pad of five layers of strong unbleached calico, wring it out of cold water, and place it on the sufferer's chest. Keep it wet. This has been known to cure very obstinate cases.

Australian Folk Medicine

In Bechuanaland they wear a ferret skin for asthma, as the animal is believed to be tenacious and difficult to kill.

African Folk Medicine

Tuberculosis

In New Zealand, the leaves of the Tikumu daisy (*Celmisia spectabilis*) were found to give relief for asthma when used as a tobacco substitute.

New Zealand/Maori Folk Medicine

Consumptive patients used to be passed three times through a circular wreath of woodbine, cut during the increase of the March moon, and let down from head to foot over the body.

Traditional English

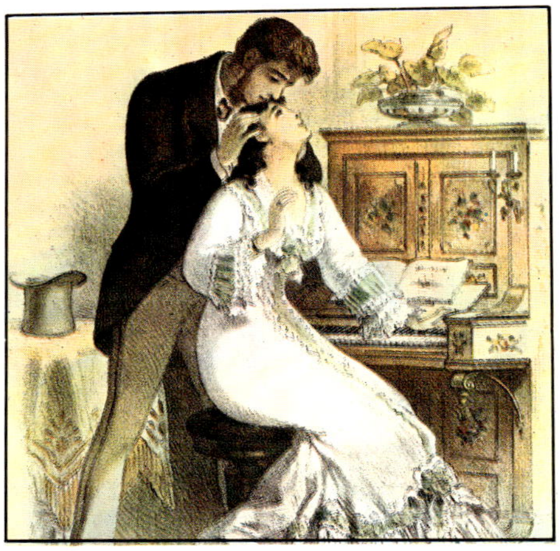

In 'La Dame aux Camélias' Dumas sentimentalized T.B.

Black nightshade leaves were steeped in water and given to people suffering from tuberculosis by the Comanche Indians. This water also expelled worms, and cured insomnia.

American Indian

Hetherd broth, made from the flesh of an adder, boiled with chicken, was considered a good cure for tuberculosis in northern England.

Traditional English

Honey and gold are recommended by the folk doctors for tuberculosis cases.

Indian Folk Medicine

The inner layer of pork lard, melted, unsalted unpasteurized butter, clear honey, and high-grade cocoa are mixed in equal parts for tuberculosis and anaemia.

Traditional Russian

Fever

Gather plenty of turds from the wild jack-rabbit, and dry them in the oven to keep for the winter in a jar. When a fever will not break, make a very strong tea of the dung and hot water, strain it, and drink it every half-hour until the sweating starts. This never fails.

American Folk Medicine, Kansas

The Maoris used an infusion of the leaves of the handsome forest tree Kohekohe (*Dysoxylum spectrabile*) as an inhalant for colds and feverish conditions.

New Zealand/Maori Folk Medicine

Dry leaves of lilac, brewed in water and drunk freely will help to bring down temperatures in fevers.

Ukrainian cure

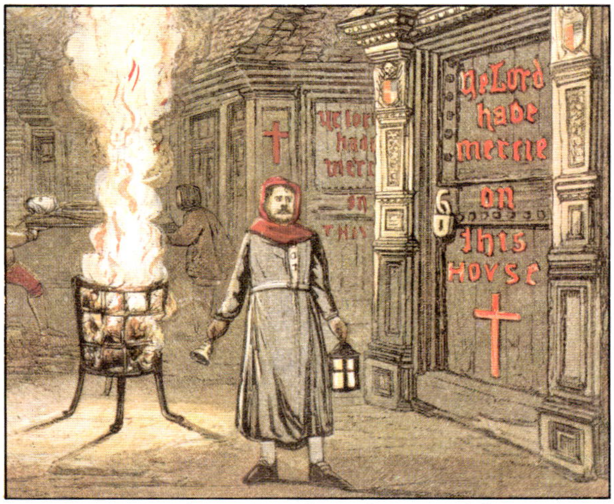

Fires were burned against plague and fever.

The leaves of the Manuka tree were used in the treatment of colds and fever.

New Zealand/Maori Folk Medicine

The Bone-set plant was widely used by early settlers, adopted from the practice of Indian doctors. It was used by the Menonimee Indians to reduce fever, also for the same by the Iroquois and Mohegans. The Iroquois also used the leaves to make a tea for a diuretic.

American Indian

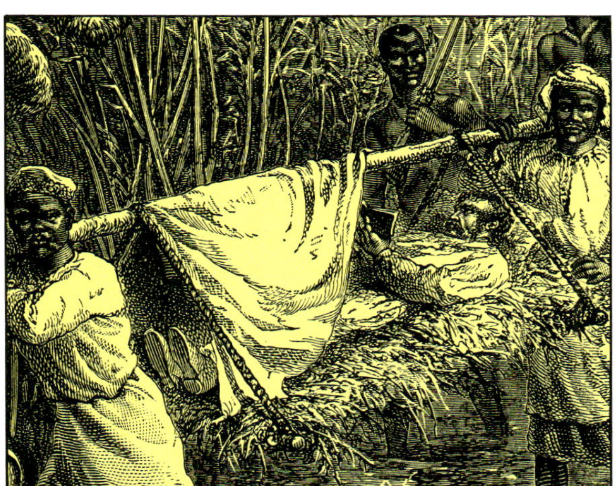

Bearers carrying the explorer Livingstone, exhausted with malarial fever.

In China, the *Ephedra* was used to induce sweating in feverish conditions. By tradition, it was always gathered and stored in the Autumn. Modern tests now show that its alkaloid content is at the highest then. The plant yields *ephedrine*, a decongestant.

Traditional Chinese

2oz pearl barley, to 5 pints of cold water. Wash the barley then put it to boil in a fresh half pint for five minutes. Then boil it again with the rest of the water until it reduces down to two pints. Strain off the liquid, which is a good cure for fevers and inflammations.

Welsh/English border

A species of *Lantana*, 'bird's brandy' or the wild sage, was among the plants brought to Africa by the Portuguese. The Africans soon established the value of these plants for native cures; the wild sage which has an action similar to quinine was used to make up a brew to help fevers and colds.

African Folk Medicine

Cholera, typhus and smallpox

Should the cholera show itself in the district, to prevent its attack take a teaspoonful of cinnamon in hot water frequently; or this simple remedy has never been known to fail; first give the patient hot water to cause vomiting, which cleanses the stomach, next toast an oatcake, this put into a pint of boiling water and drink freely.

Australian Folk Medicine

Smallpox

An old English remedy against smallpox consisted of portions of fried mice, preferably fried alive.

Traditional English

A primitive form of inoculation has long been practised among Hindus, Persians, and Chinese.

Still in north and Central Africa, this method can be found: as a cure against smallpox, a small wound is made and pus from an infected patient is rubbed in, with a chorus of prayers and incantations against the disease.

African Folk Medicine

In Japan, tradition held that people of the royal household suffering from smallpox should be laid in a red room and covered with red clothing. Even the servants all wore red. (It has been suggested that the colour is less painful to a sick person's eyes).

Japanese Folk Medicine

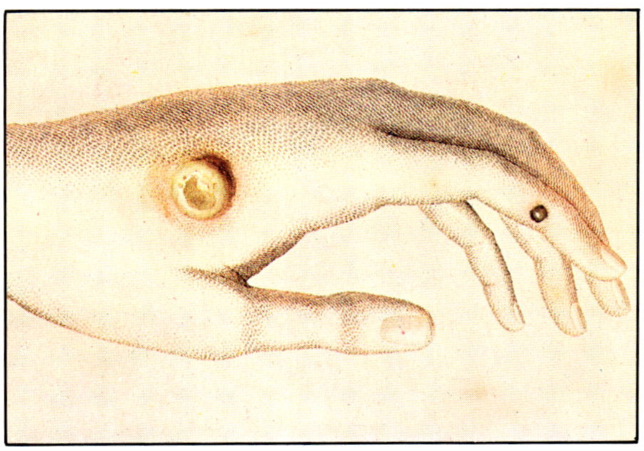

The infected pustules of smallpox.

Typhus

The *joe-pye weed* got its name from an Indian herbalist in New England who used it to cure typhus by inducing profound sweating.

American Indian

Pneumonia

Mustard powder, wetted and mixed with honey and spread on brown paper, is applied to the chest as a cure for pneumonia.

Traditional Irish

Alternatively, wool from a black sheep is covered with fried onions or sometimes mustard and egg white instead.

Traditional Irish

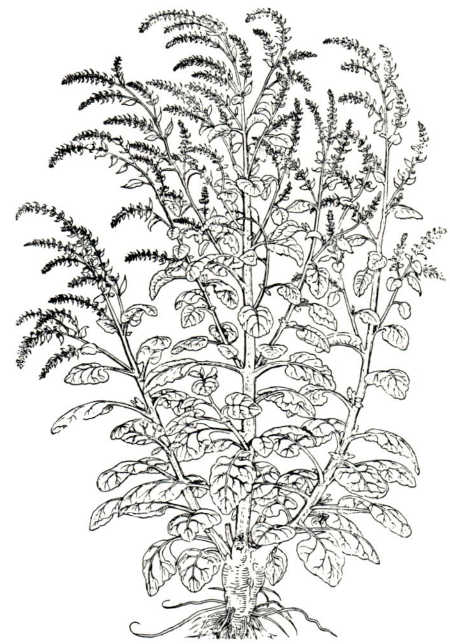

Sea beet is used in a Welsh remedy for pneumonia.

'Take a proportion of the sea beet (called in Latin *beta*) rejecting the branches and tops, and take three gallons of pure water, boiling therein; then take the beet out, letting the decoction boil, after a while remove from the fire, and let it cool to the temperature of wort, then pour it upon some fresh lees (of ale) permitting it to ferment as long as it will do so, then give it the patient for nine meals as his only drink; then take the beet and mix with butter and powdered melilot, giving it the patient to eat for nine meals, and by the help of God he will recover. It is also an excellent medicine for tertian ague'.

Traditional Welsh

Heart complaints

Take clean oats, and fry in unsalted butter till they are browned; apply to the painful part upon a cloth, and it will be most certainly cured.

Traditional Welsh

Peppermint tea, mint tea, or an infusion of hawthorn berries (squeeze berries before removing, to extract all juice) are all good tonics for those suffering from heart conditions.

Russian Folk Medicine

The folk doctors make a tea brewed from the Mexican magnolia *(Talauma mexicana)* called *yoloxochitl* or 'heart flower' in the Nahuatl language. Modern medicine has tested it and found an effect similar to digitalis, the well-known drug for heart conditions.

Mexican Folk remedy

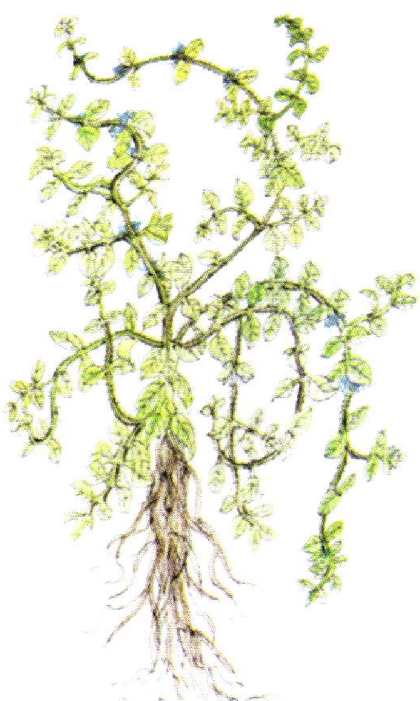

Mint is used in an infusion to alleviate heart complaints.

Skin irritations

A useful salve
$\frac{1}{2}$lb beef suet melted in a jar, 1 tablespoon of castor oil, 1 teaspoon of eucalyptus, 1 teaspoon of boracic powder. Beat all thoroughly.

Australian Folk Medicine

Sunburn
2lb of elder flowers simmered in 2lb of hog's lard until crisp, then sieved out. The fat is good for sunburn.

Australian Folk Medicine

2oz of lettuce juice, 2drs of Eau de Cologne, 2oz of distilled vinegar, 4oz of elder flower water, well mixed. Dab the skin frequently on irritated part.

Welsh/English border

Skin complaints, ranging from prurigo and lichen to scabies, are treated with papaya fruit.
(Papaya contains valuable enzymes, very good for the skin).

Mexican Folk Medicine

The most severe skin diseases were treated by the Maoris by bathing in a hot decoction of the bark of the Hinau tree.

New Zealand/Maori Folk Medicine

A cure for the itch is to take the inner bark of the elder tree, boil it in vinegar, and dab the liquid on the area. This also helps to take away scabs.

Traditional English

Shingles
Shingles can be cured by applying zinc ointment: the person making the cure should say ten Our Fathers and ten Hail Marys.

Traditional Irish

Another cure is to apply fasting spittle and make the sign of a cross with a wedding ring over the spot.

Traditional Irish and English

Scabies
Scabies are treated by eating young alligators and washing the skin with urine.

Mexican Folk Medicine

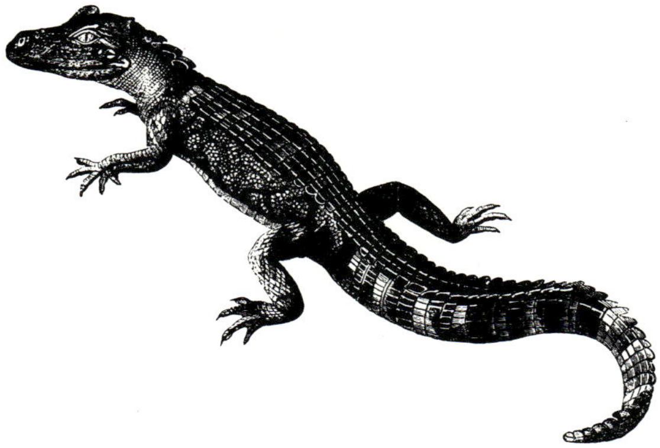

Boils and blisters
Worms are believed to be the source of many illnesses, like boils. A poultice of the boiled roots of the comfrey plant is applied in the belief that worms hate the smell and the one in the boil will come out.

Traditional Irish

Dock tea is a long-established remedy for applying to boils.

Traditional English

To cure boils the Maoris made a drawing poultice from the pith of the Pargon tree, commonly called the silver tree fern.

New Zealand/Maori Folk Medicine

Toad cure
The Chinese used to have a great belief in the curative powers of the toad, as it is one of the 'five poisons', the others being snake, scorpion, centipede and black spider. It used to be the custom to sprinkle wine on the floor on the fifth day of the fifth month to get rid of these pests. Toad was used to make plasters for boils, abscesses etc. (It contains adrenalin and bufagin, which acts similarly to digitalis). Traditionally, the secretion from the toad was collected in a strange way. A toad is surrounded with mirrors on all sides. It becomes uncomfortable, and secretes juice from a gland between its eyes, on its head. This juice is used for the plaster.

Chinese traditional medicine

For cuts or boils, the folk doctor applies hot mango leaf with a paste of wheat flour, or alternatively a cowdung poultice. Sometimes these treatments are piled up in successive layers!

North India Remedy

An old cure is to put a poultice on a boil for three days and nights, then to put the poultice cloths into the coffin of a dead man.

Transference cure

The flowers of beans and fenugreek, mixed with honey, are good for boils and bruises.

Traditional English

The skin of a boiled egg, applied wet, is a good boil remedy.

Australian Folk Medicine

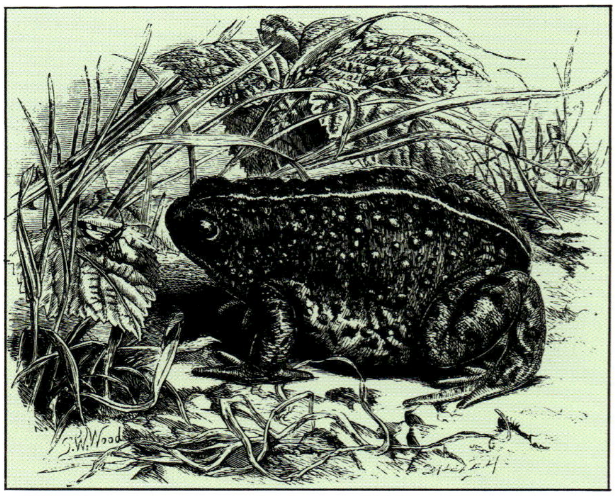

Toads were used for boils.

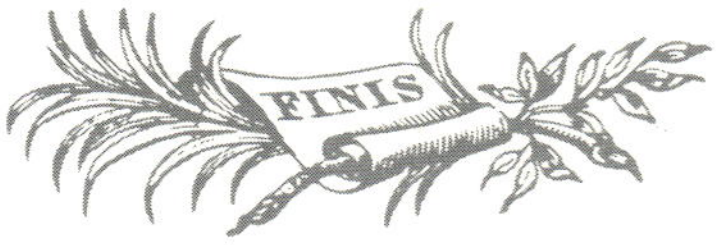

Sores, burns and bites

Running sores
Powdered vervain, (root and leaf) should be applied to running sores, boiled with fresh butter to make a little wax. Strain it and apply it.
Traditional Welsh

The touch of a dead man is a traditional cure for running sores.
Transference cure

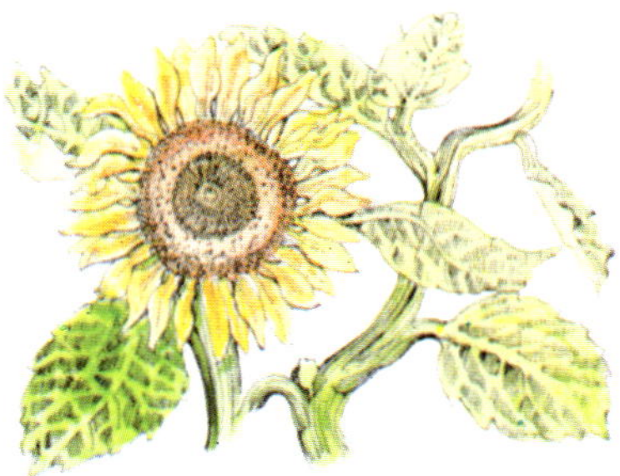

Sunflower. The root is mashed to draw blisters.

The Ojibwa Indians used to take the crushed root of the sunflower (*Helianthus annuus*) and apply it mashed in a wet dressing for drawing blisters.
American Indian

Burns
To cure running sores, the Maoris used the inner bark of the Pukatea (*Laurelia novae zelandiae.*) The inner bark was stripped off and steeped in hot water. It was also used to cure blisters.
New Zealand/Maori Folk Medicine

1 part beeswax by weight, four parts mutton fat, heated together in a double saucepan. Sometimes camomile flowers may be added. When needed, heat the grease and apply as a thick dressing to the burn. Or better, soak bandages in the mixture while it is being prepared and allow to harden and keep for use as required. Use two or more thicknesses, and a bandage to keep it in place.
Traditional Irish

A chant to cure sores and burns:
Here come I to cure a burnt sore,
If the dead knew what the living endure,
The burnt sore would burn no more.
Shetland Islands

Roast a dozen eggs, stone hard, then take out the yolk and put in a frying pan, fry them till they become an ointment and strain; anoint the injured part with the same, then take a bladder, spread mucilage of lime twigs thereon, and apply to the injured part.
Traditional Welsh

Australian settlers soon used the eucalyptus tree as a general cure-all; the leaves themselves were bound over blisters and burns.
Traditional Australian

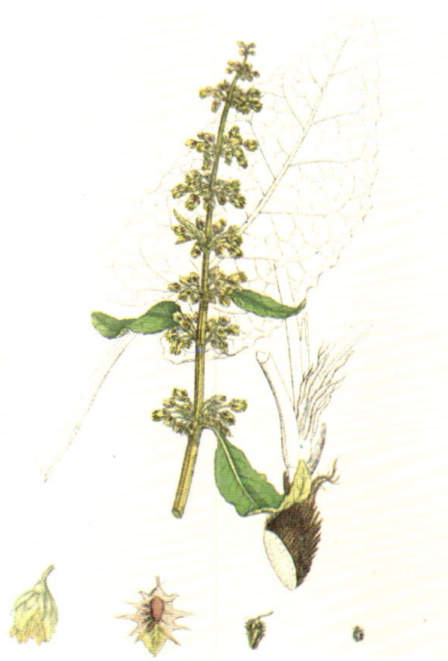

Dock leaves soothe nettle stings.

Stings and bites
Dock leaves are the acknowledged remedy for nettle stings in all parts of the British Isles. Here is an Irish chant to accompany the rubbing of a dock leaf on the affected part:
Dockin, Dockin in and out,
Take the sting of the nettle out.
another:

Neanntog a thoit me,
Biolar sraide leighis me
(a nettle burned me, dock cure me)

Bee stings
Bee stings are traditionally cured by applying a blue bag (used for rinsing clothes) to take away the smarting pain.

Traditional Irish

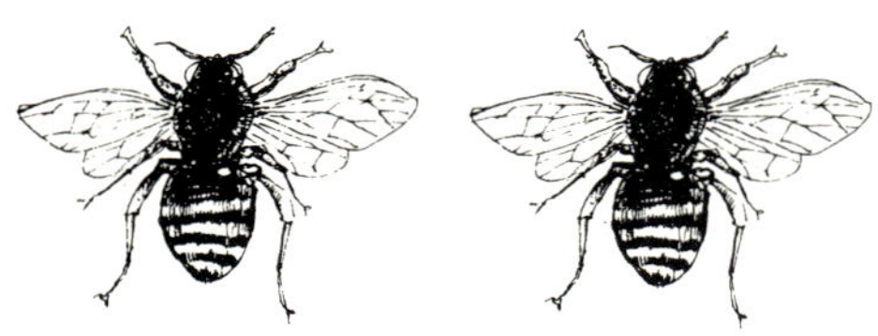

Spider bites
Take nine cloves of garlic and peel carefully, a spoonful of treacle, a quart of new strong ale, mix these together and give them to the patient to drink freely at the same time cover him with an abundance of clothes so that he may perspire well. If he can retain this position for an hour he will escape even though the integument had become mottled. This medicament is also useful for a person bitten by an adder.

Traditional Welsh

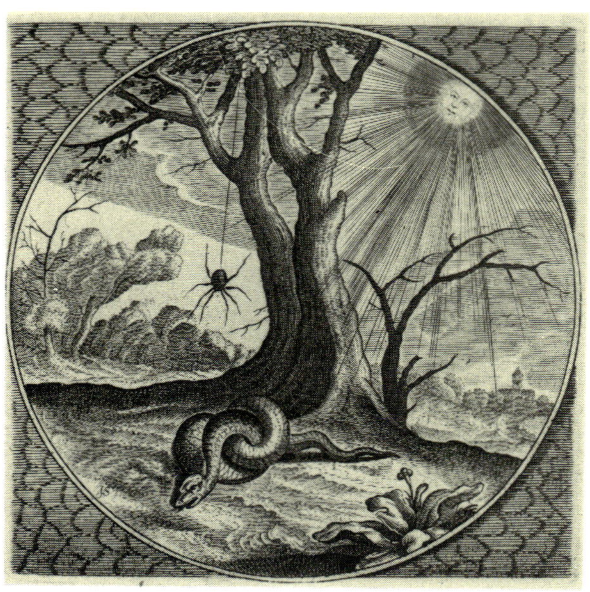

Pimpernel and other speckled plants, those looking like viper's skin, are good for use in cures against bites or stings.

Sympathetic cure

Dog bite
Mad dog bites are best treated with the seeds of nettles.

Traditional English

Scorpion bites
Run fast and find three kinds of leaves, one jagged (like the dandelion) one round, and one long. Crush them in your hand and rub them hard over the bitten place. Rub rub *rub*.

Provençal French

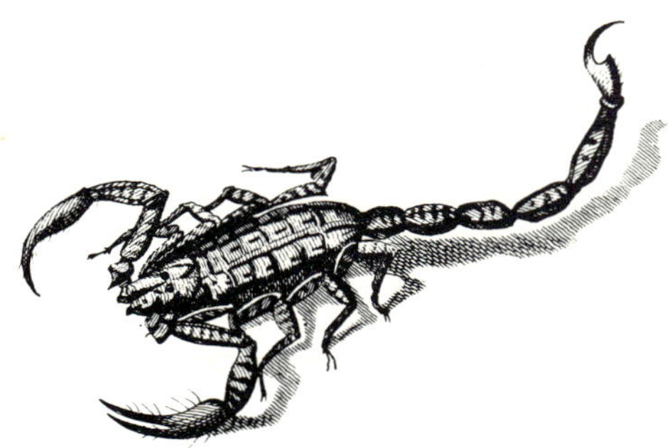

Rattlesnake bite
Leaves of the white ash were used by all tribes of Indians as a cure for rattlesnake bites. Hunters soon learned to stuff their boots with them.

American Indian

Cape cure
In the Cape, a folk cure for a snake bite is to pluck feathers from a chicken, make a cut in its body and hold the wound over the bite until the poison is 'drawn out' of the bite and the chicken dies.

Transference cure: African Folk Medicine

Almost the same practice has been recorded in old Devonshire, but here the chicken is killed and the bird's open stomach is thrust against the sufferer's wound.

Transference cure

Corns and chilblains

Corns

A handful of ivy leaves put to steep in a pint of vinegar in a tightly corked bottle should be left to stand for 48 hours. Pour off the liquid leaving the sediment and leaves behind, and keep it tightly corked again. Use it to bathe corns, but apply carefully to just the corn, not to soft skin.

Traditional Irish

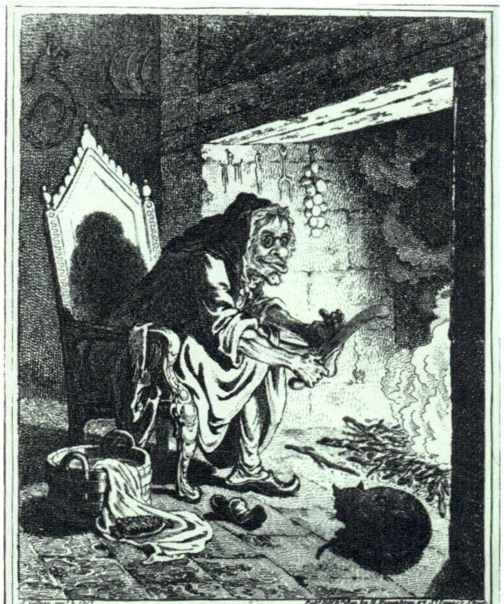

COMFORT to the CORNS.

The New Zealand Kawakawa or Pepper tree has many medicinal uses. To cure corns a poultice of the boiled leaves would draw out the corn.

New Zealand/Maori Folk Medicine

Pour two teaspoons of vinegar into an egg cup, and drop into it a piece of copper wire. Let it stand for a couple of days, then use as follows: just paint the corns with the vinegar-soaked wire once or twice a day. The corns become soft, and can be lifted out without soreness. (Alternatively, soak pennies for 48 hours in a strong vinegar and apply the resulting solution). Or put equal parts of soda and soap on a thick rag, bind the corn till morning.

Australian Folk Medicine

Pare closely then apply bruised ivy leaves daily. The corn will drop out within a fortnight. Corns or sore feet can be eased by soaking them in water in which oatmeal has been boiled.

Welsh/English border

Chilblains

Chilblains can be treated with equal parts of methylated spirits and separated milk, mixed together. This is applied to the chilblains night and morning.

Australian Folk Medicine

A mustard liniment is considered very good. Or, bathing with water potatoes have boiled in, as hot as possible.

Australian Folk Medicine

Take the peel of cucumbers and dry it. When needed, soften the inside part with water and apply to the chilblains.

Russian Folk Medicine

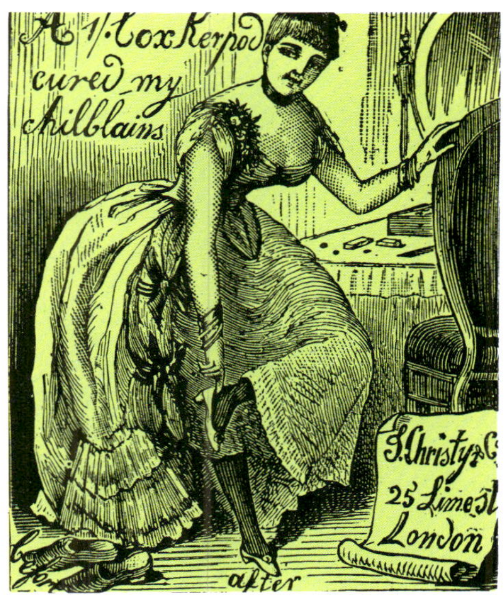

Wounds and bleeding

Bleeding

An adder's tongue, chopped up, was considered good for cuts.

Lincolnshire remedy

Take the ashes of snake's skin, and keep them carefully, for they are the most precious application which any human tongue can order. Let the first instance at hand suffice: whoever has a fresh wound, let him cover it with a little of this ash, and it will heal it in three days.

Traditional Welsh

To heal a wound: Take yellow wax, melt on a slow fire, and take bruised cumin seed, mix with the molten wax, then stir these ingredients with a stirrer until cold. Apply this as a plaster to the wound.

Traditional Welsh

The vervain, known as the 'holy herb' was one of the sacred plants of the Druids, and has a long history as a healing plant, as the rhyme explains:

All hail, thou holy herb, vervin,
Growing on the ground;
On the Mount of Calvary
There wast thou found;
Thou helpest many a grief,
And staunchest many a wound,
In the name of sweet Jesu,
I lift thee from the ground.

Traditional English

Fill your mouth with tender guava leaves and chew them to a soft paste, and then put them on the cut.

Tahiti and Central America

The Maoris used the varieties of Puwha (sow thistle) as an effective wound dressing. The leaves were crushed and bound over the wound, and have proved to contain a blood purifier.

New Zealand/Maori Folk Medicine

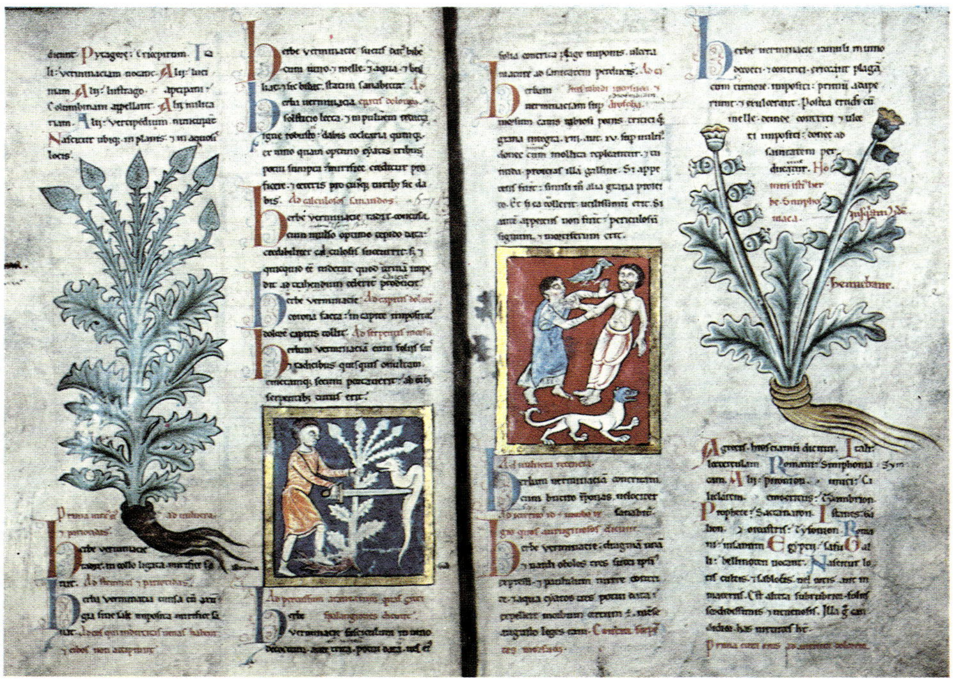

Vervain, the 'holy herb' is shown on the left of this manuscript.

To stop bleeding, apply the cobweb.

Traditional English

In China, traditionally they used spagnum moss over wounds. It does contain medically-established antiseptic properties.

Chinese Folk Medicine

The Thompson Indians of British Columbia used to use valerian in their medicine bags. The fresh roots were pulverized and applied to wounds.

British Columbia

Polynesians used papaya on wounds to help heal them. Papaya contains valuable enzymes which are very good for the skin.

Polynesia

Water distilled from frog spawn, gathered in March is good for wounds and bleeding. Warm a teaspoonful and then drop it into the wound.

Traditional English

Balsam from the sweet gum was boiled with water and the hot liquid was applied to wounds. (This is a native American tree, related to the *Oriental Liquidambar*. The gum from it was recognized by the US Pharmacopoiea up until 1926).

Traditional American

The heated leaves of the Kawakawa tree produced a juice with which the Maoris dressed badly infected wounds.

New Zealand/Maori Folk Medicine

The common plantain is macerated and applied to a wound, then covered with a bandage. The medical virtues of the plantain are long established.

Traditional English

It used to be believed that bleeding could be stopped by tying a thread around the patient's thumb. This fastened the soul in the body.

Traditional Scottish

The ancient Chinese used to soak lemons in brine, and use the juice on wounds. There would be some real medical value in this remedy as Vitamin C plays an important part in the formation of collagen, necessary for holding skin cells together.

Chinese Folk Medicine

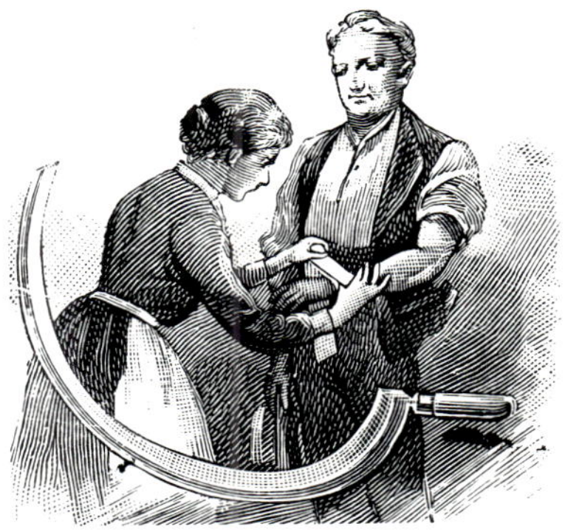

Warts

Rub the warts daily with a radish, or with the juice of marigold flowers, or with a piece of raw meat.

Welsh/English border

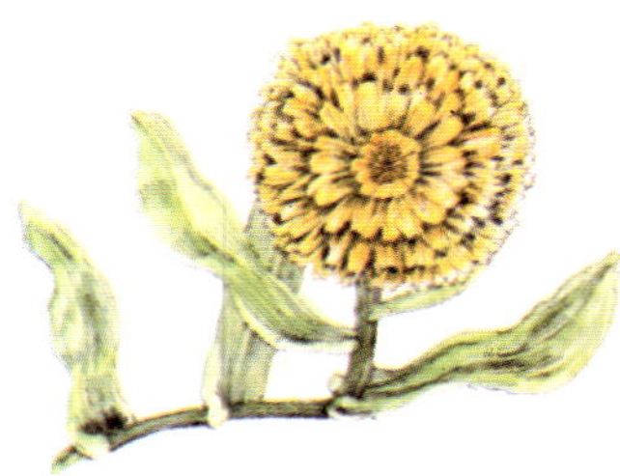

Marigold flowers for warts.

Rub with a raw potato, and bury the potato in clay. Repeat the next day with another bit of potato to be sure. Touching the coat of a man who never saw his own father will do it.
Or apply the milky sap from a dandelion flower.

Traditional Irish

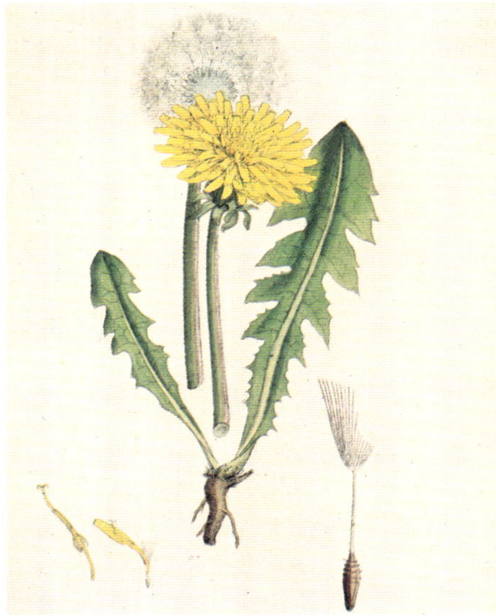

Rub dandelion sap on warts.

Rub warts with a black snail, then impale it on a thorn tree. As the snail dries and withers, so do the warts.

Transference cure

Killing a toad used to be thought to cause warts in New England.

American Folk Medicine

Rub the wart with a strip of bacon, and slip it under the bark of an ash tree, to make it disappear.

Traditional English

Rub the warts with a cinder, tie it up in paper, and leave it at some crossroads. Whoever goes and picks up the parcel and unwraps it, gets the warts.

Transference cure

Prick the wart with a gooseberry thorn passed through a wedding ring.

Traditional English

Fasting spittle is good for warts.

Traditional English

Wet a forefinger with your saliva, and point it in the direction of a passing funeral three times, saying, "My wart goes with you."

Traditional English

Count the warts, put an equal number of stones in a bag and bury it.

Lincolnshire remedy

Rub the wart with a piece of stolen beef, then bury the meat.

Scottish remedy

The milky juice of the Mexican poppy (*Argemone mexicana*) is applied locally to cure warts.

African Folk Medicine

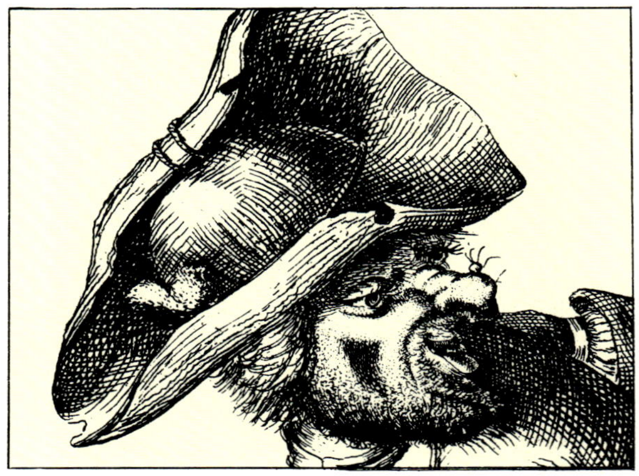

FINIS

Ear and headaches

Headaches

North American Indians used to cure headaches with a potion made from the testes of the beaver, bottled in spirit. *Castoreum* is still officially used in some foreign pharmacopoieas, in this century.

American Indian

The Meskwakis Indians made a tea from the root and bark of the American elder (*Sambucus canadensis*) to treat headaches and encourage the expulsion of phlegm.

American Indian

A simple cure for a headache is to put salt on the tongue, then wash it down with warm water.

American Folk Medicine

'2 ounses of Rubbarb leaves sliced, 1 ounse of Jensit's bark in powder, 2 ounces of sugar candy, 2 drams of Juniper Berris, Sinamon & nutmeg of each a dram: a Quart of strong wine infuse it in.'

American Traditional

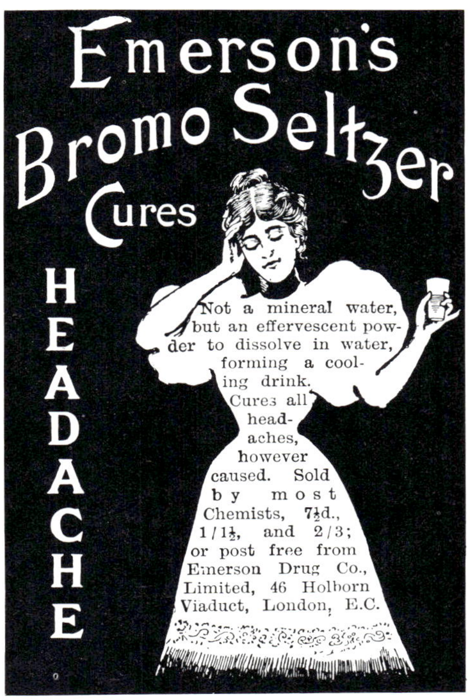

Earache

Take a loaf of wheaten bread (ground through) hot from the oven, divide it in two, and apply to both ears as hot as it can be borne, bind, and thus produce perspiration, and by the help of God you will be cured.

Traditional Welsh

Put salt in a frying pan, heat it, and place in a bag to make a pillow. It gives tremendous relief for earache.

Australian Folk Medicine

Toothache

It is a widespread belief, all over the world, that toothache is caused by a worm gnawing into the tooth – as far apart places as China, Europe, and Australasia have cures based on this idea.

The two varieties of Horopito (Pepper trees) in New Zealand were commonly called 'Maori Pain Killers'. The leaves are chewed to cure toothache.

New Zealand/Maori Folk Medicine

'Take distilled water of red roses, a small portion of beeswax, and a little fresh butter, say an equal quantity of each; let the ingredients be mixed together in a dish upon embers, then let a linen cloth be dipped therein, and applied to the affected jaw as hot as it can be borne.

Traditional Welsh

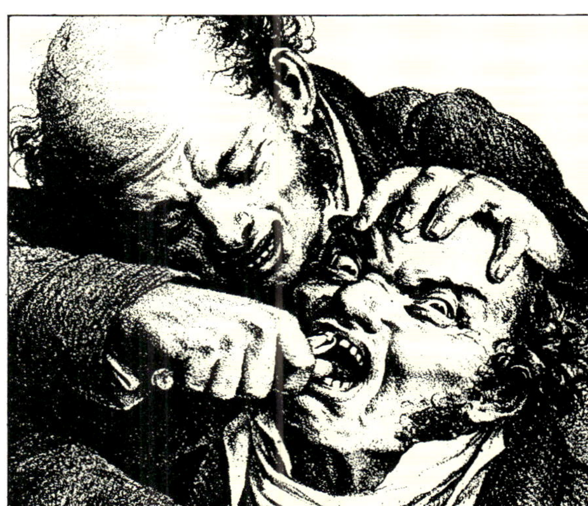

In Russia, a favoured remedy is a hot infusion of sage leaves, used as a mouth rinse.

Russian Folk Medicine

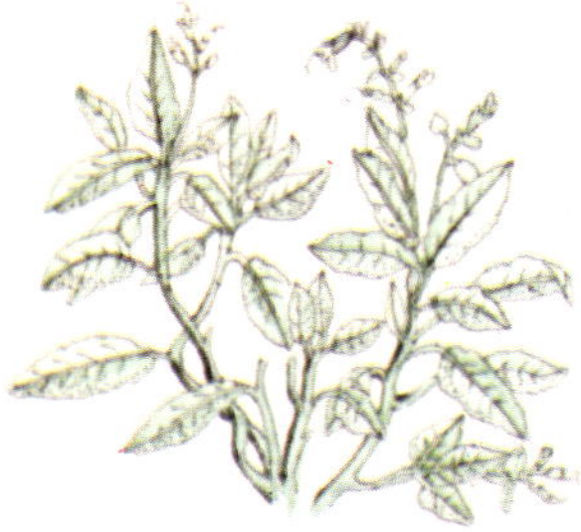

Sage cures toothache.

'A good old-fashioned cure, which succeeds often when everything else fails. Dip a small piece of strong brown paper in whisky, sprinkle it with pepper, and apply to the face where the pain is. Cover with a flannel bandage. It does not blister the skin.

Australian Folk Medicine

Henbane, orpin and vervain green, cut into beads to make a teething ring. Soak in wine with powdered coral.

Traditional English

Eye complaints

Styes

One hair from a black cat, pulled out of its tail on the first night of the new moon and applied to a stye nine times, will cure it.

Traditional American

Try a teaspoon of black tea in a tiny bag, just moistened with boiling water, and apply as a poultice. Keep this on the eye all night, and the stye should be gone in the morning. Take also a dose of purgative medicine, such as Epsom Salts, with a squeeze of lemon in it.

Australian remedy

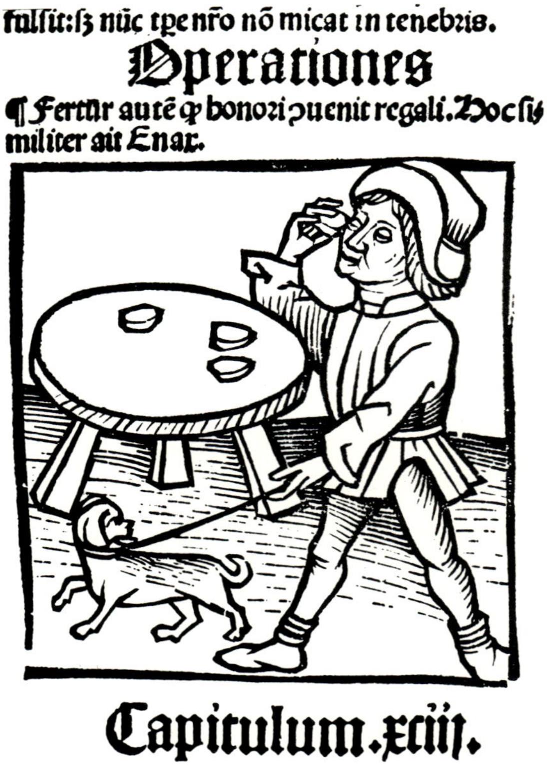
fulsit:sz nūc tpe nr̄o nō micat in tenebris.
Operationes
¶ Fertur autē q bonori ꝯuenit regali. Hoc si militer ait Enax.
Capitulum.xciij.

Rub a stye with a tom cat's tail.

Traditional English

Fasting spittle rubbed on each morning will cure them or rub them with a wedding ring.

Australian Folk Medicine

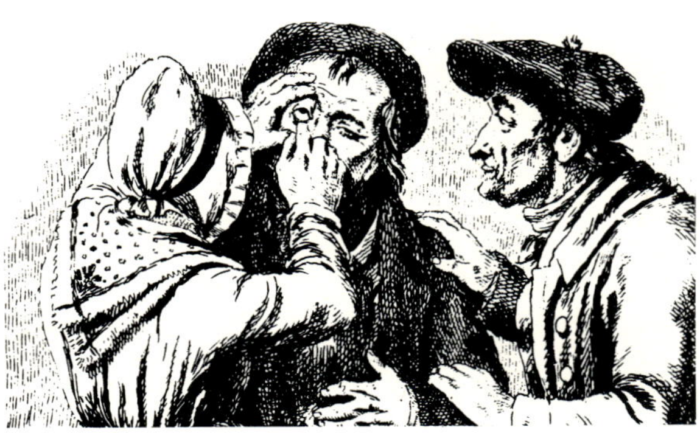

Eye strain

For tired eyes, compresses of raw grated potatoes, apples, or cucumbers are to be recommended, and the flower eyebright is also good.

Russian Folk Medicine

Sore eyes were treated by the Maoris by boiling the leaves of the Makomato (wineberry) tree, and bathing the eyes with the liquid. They also soaked the bark in cold water for eye troubles.

New Zealand/Maori Folk Medicine

Insomnia

The Meskwaki Indians used to gather hops and use them to stuff pillows, which were then used for sedative purposes or to induce sleep.

American Indian

Eat two or three raw onions, or onion jelly: shred two or three good-sized onions in a little stock, and stew until tender. Add a squeeze of fresh lemon juice, then add enough water to make a soup. Boil for ten minutes, then add seasonings, and a small piece of butter.

Welsh/English border

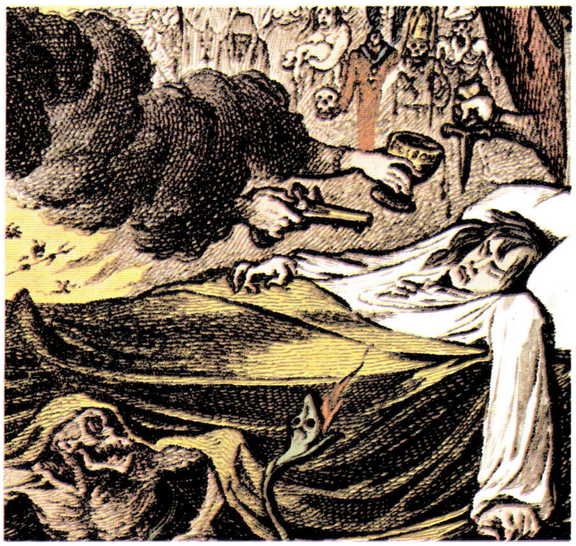

A Siberian sleeping potion:

Valerian infusion	2 parts
Apple vinegar	1 part
Clear honey	3 parts
Vodka or gin	2 parts
Hot milk	2 parts

(Valerian infusion is made by putting 1 teaspoon of the root to one glass of water. Infuse for one hour, then strain. If bought as a tincture, then use 10 to 20 drops).

Russian Folk Medicine

Rheumatism

Carry a potato in the pocket, raw, as a charm against rheumatism; or failing that a chestnut, either begged or stolen.

Traditional English

For rheumatism the Maoris used a pulp of the leaves of the Kawakawa (Pepper tree). The pulp was made with hot water, and the resulting mash held against the painful area.

New Zealand/Maori Folk Medicine

Another Maori cure for rheumatism, arthritis and sciatic pain is derived from the Harakeke plant New Zealand Hemp. Used for a variety of domestic purposes, the rheumatism cure was made by boiling the broad base of the leaves and rubbing the warm liquid on the affected limbs.

New Zealand/Maori Folk Medicine

A nutmeg carried in the pocket is a protection against rheumatism.

Traditional English

Black slugs steeped in tea will ease the pains, if the decoction is used as a liniment applied to the limbs.

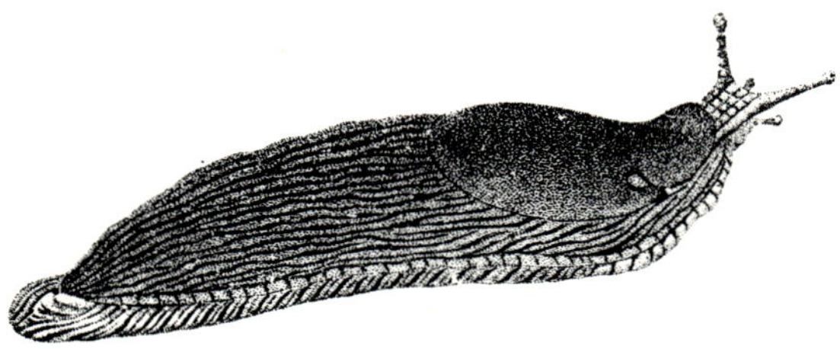

Pig fat rubbed into stiff joints will ease the pain.

Try a poultice of boiled seaweed for rheumatic joints.

Willow bark tea was an old Indian remedy for stiff joints and rheumatism; according to the *Doctrine of Signatures*, the supple swaying movement of the tree's branches proved that it was good for this ailment. The bark actually contains something similar to aspirin base, salicylic acid.

American Indian

To make a poultice to soothe the pains of rheumatism or any other:
Pick stinging nettles and young oak leaves, chop them, put them into a fine handkerchief or piece of gauze, sprinkle them with sulpur, and bind firmly over the painful spot.

Swiss traditional remedy

Cider vinegar makes a good rub for the relief of rheumatism, arthritis, and even varicose veins in both man and beast.

American remedy, New England

Another, is to carry the right forefoot of a hare.

Traditional English

Cod liver oil has been used as a remedy by many different sea-side communities, such as the Lapps, and the Eskimos.

Arctic remedy

The touch of a dead man's limbs is supposed to cure rheumatism.

Traditional Irish

Bee stings have long been considered a good folk remedy for rheumatism. (This is possibly to do with formic acid present in their venom).

Traditional English

In the Urals, salt baths in oaken vats were prescribed, lasting ten to twenty minutes as hot as possible, together with the taking of enemas. Sometimes bran was added to the bath, or birch leaf, or pine needles.

Russian Folk Medicine

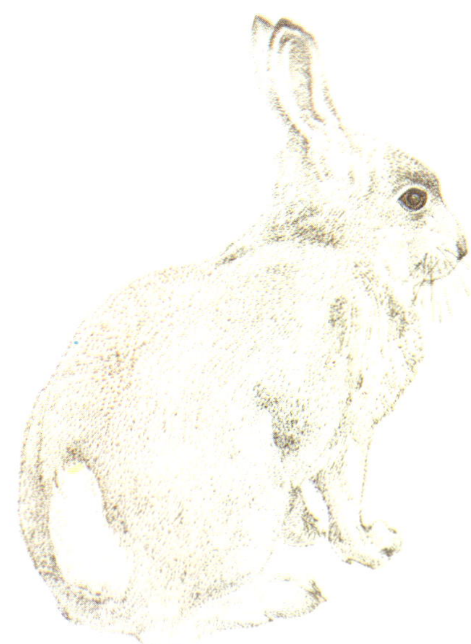

FINIS

Aches and pains

Cramp can be avoided by keeping a piece of sulphur tucked under your pillow, or make a sulphur band by sewing a bit into a garter.

Scottish remedies

'For all kinds of hurtful aches in whatever way they come:
Get parsley, plantain, daisy, garlic, and grains of Paradise, pound well in a mortar, strain and take the juice in ale. If the patient can obtain beef, he should not eat it when he recovers'.

Traditional Welsh

Sprains

A sprain can be cured by going to a weaver, who will tie a weaver's knot around it, or a piece of red thread. (This is only for injury to a joint without fracture or dislocation.)

Traditional English

Eelskin is considered good for sprains of the limbs – presumably because of the lithe and slippery nature of the fish.

Traditional Irish

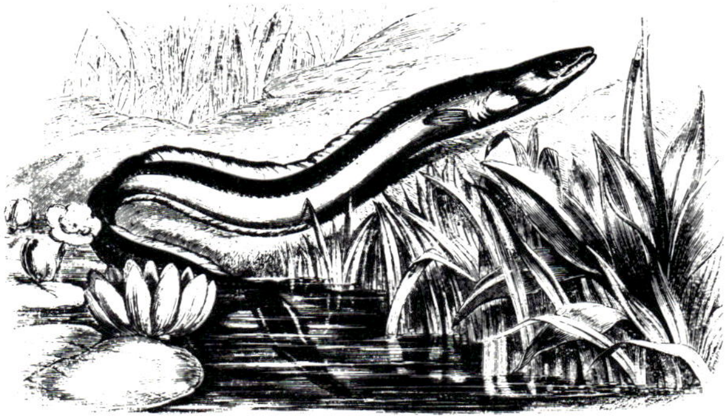

A sprained ankle can be cured with an alcohol made from rotting pears: it helps to keep down the swelling.

American Folk Medicine

Housemaid's knee

Housemaid's knee used to be cured with a poultice of sugar damped and wrapped in strong brown paper.

Traditional Irish

Backache

The Cherokees drank a tea of the roots of the spikenard (*Aralia racemosa*) for relief of backache; this was soon adopted as a remedy by the early settlers of the Great Smoky mountains. The root was in the official National Formulary from 1916 to 1965, to be used for rheumatism. It contains a saponin called *aralin*.

American Indian

The Indians, and then the settlers, widely used witchhazel (*Hamamelis virginiana*). The Menominees of Wisconsin boiled the leaves and rubbed the liquid into the legs of sportsmen to ease their legs for racing. A decoction of the boiled twigs was also good for backache. (This too was in the National Formulary from 1916 to 1965. It is still used to relieve inflammations and bruises.)

American Indian

It used to be held that people born breech presentation (bottom first) had the 'cure' for sprains, lumbago and rheumatism.

Traditional English

Gout

A heap of ants boiled in water is a good remedy for gout. (Sympathetic cure, as ants are lively and wriggly.)

Traditional English

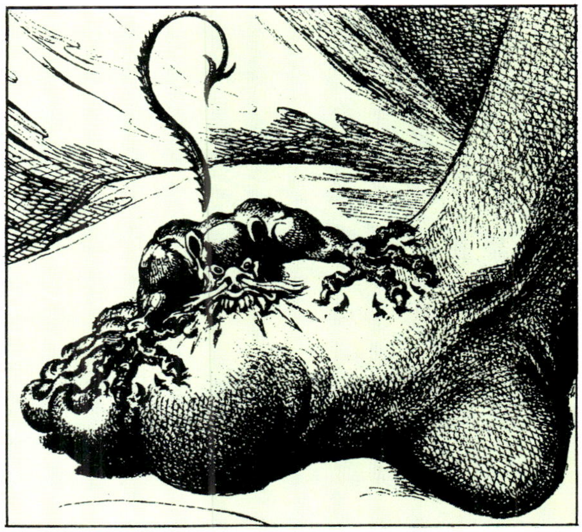

The gout is both painful and distorts the foot.

A German remedy for gout is to take hold of an oak, or of a young shoot already felled, and to repeat these words:

'Oak-shoot, I to thee complain,
All the torturing gout plagues me;
I cannot go for it,
Thou canst stand it.
The first bird that flies above thee,
To him give it in his flight,
Let him take it with him in the air.'

German Folk Medicine

Lumbago

Mix 2oz of mustard with ½ pint of spirits of wine and 2 drs of camphor. Stand for two to three days, corked in a bottle. Strain and keep closely bottled.

Welsh/English border

Arthritis

Herb dealers prescribe a tea with a finely chopped root of the yam as a cure for arthritis; modern scientists are now investigating yams for the yield of *botogenin* – a starter for synthesizing cortizone.

Mexican Folk remedy

An Aztec cure for arthritic hands was to plunge them deep into an anthill.

Mexican Folk remedy

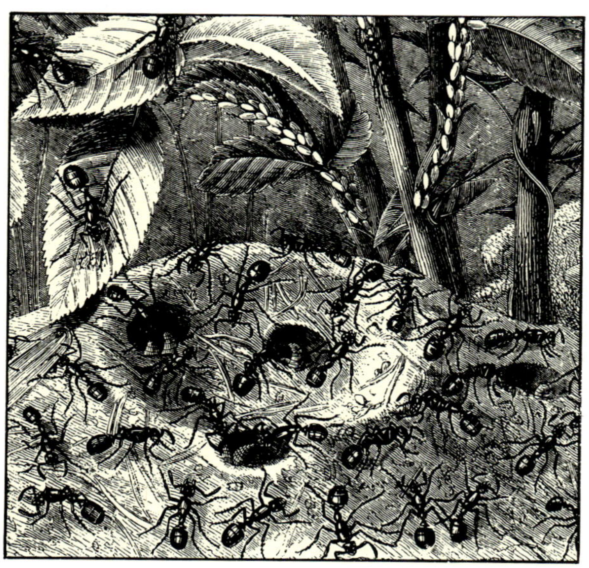

Anthill baths are recommended for arthritis: the ants are boiled then added whole with the water to a hot bath. The formic acid so released is a good pain reliever.

Russian Folk Medicine

Epilepsy and fits

It must be remembered that knowledge of mental diseases is confined to recent developments in medicine. This area of folk medicine is the most out of date, and often, barbarous. Definitions of insanity, or understanding of the causes of quite unrelated conditions, such as epilepsy, were unknown until this century. At the same time, many native doctors or herbalists have hit upon a local plant to treat these various conditions, which modern science has proved to be beneficial, and occasionally, irreplaceable.

Epilepsy

The Mexican magnolia (*Talauma mexicana*) yields a syrup from its blossom, used for epileptic cases, and heart diseases. The root is supposed to have an action similar to digitalis.

Mexican Folk Medicine

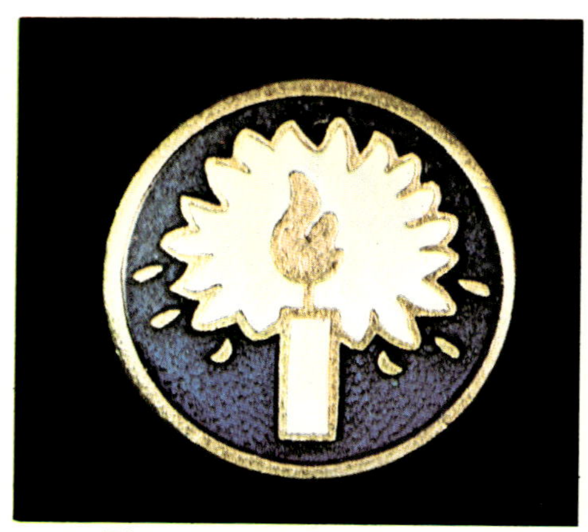

This distinctive lapel badge is worn by British epileptics.

'Fear water' used to be a remedy for epilepsy. This could be produced by a woman wearing a bottle round her neck during intercourse, where orgasm is simultaneous. The water could be used for a young girl suffering from hysteria also. It was drunk in small doses throughout the day.

Russian Folk Medicine

A concoction made from a whole swallow was considered a good cure for hysteria, palsy, and kidney trouble. The stone of a swallow could cure epilepsy and blindness (preferably taken from the body on a Wednesday.)

Traditional English

The dried body of a frog worn in a silk bag round the neck would avert epilepsy or any kind of fit.

Traditional English

A handful of earth off a fresh grave, gathered at midnight, is a good cure for fits.

Traditional English

Powder of a man's bones, especially the skull, is good for epilepsy.

Traditional English

Nine pieces of elder cut from between two knots is a good amulet for epilepsy.

Traditional English

Three drops of blood from a black cat's tail will cure epilepsy.

American Folk Medicine

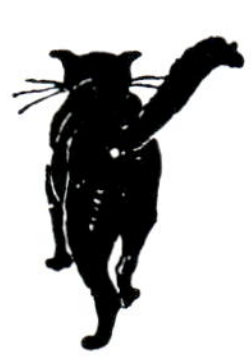

Painkillers

Throughout South America, the Indians have always used the various local narcotic plants, *coca* in the Andes, *peyote* in Mexico and also the *ololiuqui* (the morning glory). These are variously used for insomnia, for insanity, or as painkillers. Herbwomen in Mexico still pound the seeds of the *ololiuqui* to make a salve to numb pains. The Incas used to perform 'ritual surgery' on patients, using various species of *Datura* to produce a numbing effect. (In the Andes, a tree variety is found, *Datura fastuosa*.)

South American Folk Medicine

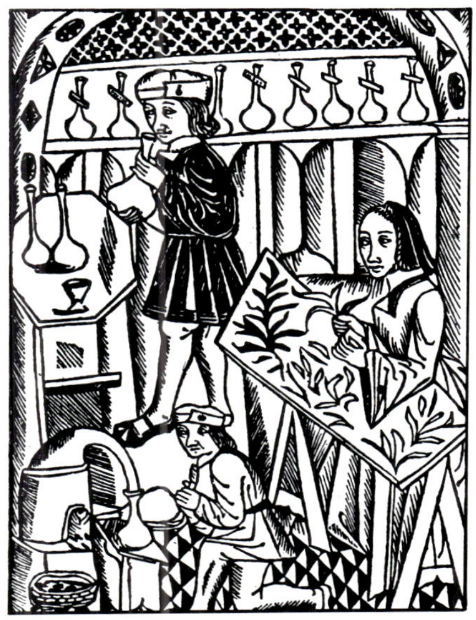

In North Africa, the *catha* plant is used to deaden pain, for those taking part in ordeal ceremonies.

African Folk Medicine

A mixture of hops and camomile flowers made into an infusion and used as a poultice will deaden pain.

Traditional English

Beauty treatments

Skin lotion
Half fill a bottle with oatmeal, and top it up with water. Shake up the mixture regularly, inverting the bottle. Soak for 24 hours. Pour off the water and use it as a skin lotion. This is very good for cleansing the pores.

Traditional Irish

Face pack
Buttermilk and oatmeal will make a good face pack.

Traditional Irish

Freckle treatment
To remove freckles, wash the face with buttermilk, in which silver weed (*Potentilla anserina*) has been steeped for nine days.

Traditional Scottish

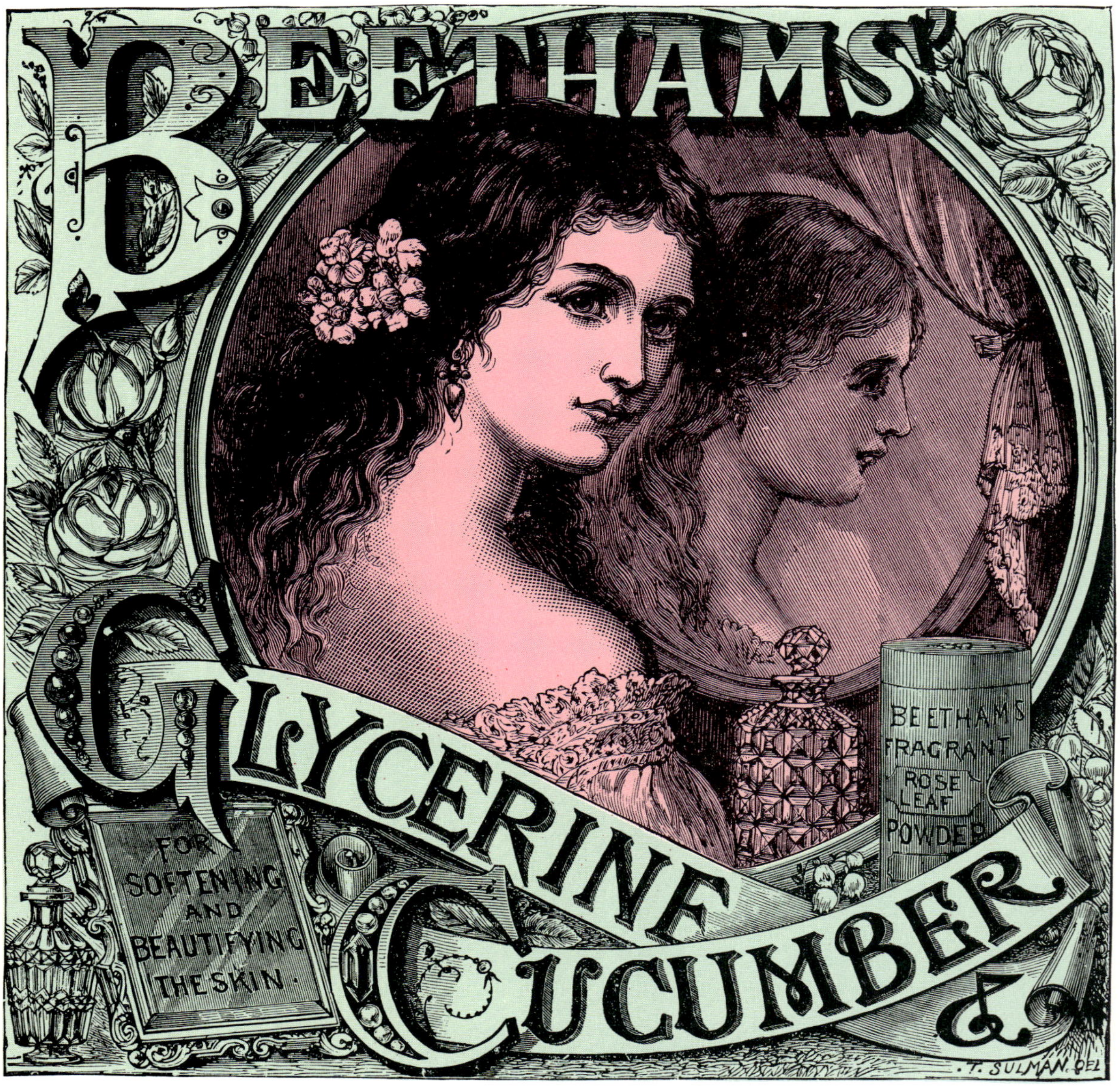

The elder flower made into a water, is a good remedy for freckles, and soothes skin irritations.

Traditional English

Camomile lotion

Place 5 or 6 dried flowers of camomile in a bowl and pour a half-pint of boiling water over them. Cover the bowl and allow to steep for 10 or 12 minutes. When the lotion has slightly cooled, sponge it on the skin with a small pad of cotton wool. This is good for enlarged pores and toning up relaxed muscles. It can also be used as a hair tonic.

Welsh/English border

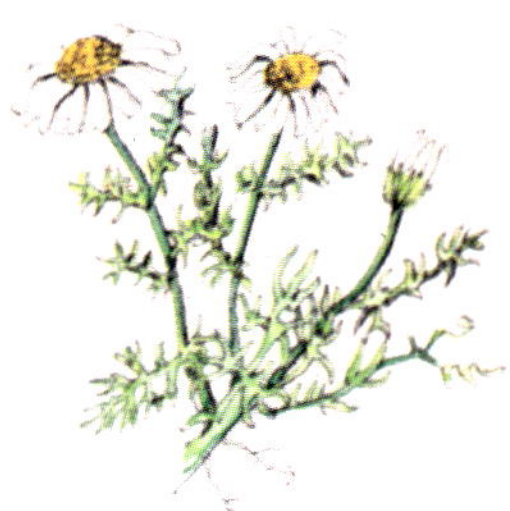

Camomile flowers.

Hairwash

Peach kernels boiled in vinegar make an excellent wash for the hair.

Traditional English

Grey hair tonic

1 dessertspoon of salt, four dessertspoons of good brandy: put in a bottle and shake up for 5 minutes. Although a sediment of salt will remain in the bottom of the bottle, it is quite ready for use, and must not be shaken again. Rub well into the roots of the hair twice a week.

Australian Folk Medicine

For dandruff

Two tablespoons of the dry herb, self-heal or wild burnet (*Prunella vulgaris*) is put into 1 quart of water and boiled for 20 minutes. Strain the liquid and use as a hair wash without soap. Allow it to dry on the hair. Repeat this for a few days.

Russian Folk medicine

To make the hair beautifully glossy Maori women poured boiling water over the young leaf tips of the Ngaio tree, and when cool the liquid was rubbed in the hair as a rinse after a shampoo. It also treats dandruff.

New Zealand/Maori Folk Medicine

A skin softener

Fresh cucumbers are washed and cut into small slices, and placed in a bottle. This is filled with vodka or dilute alcohol (50% strength), and kept in the sun or in a warm place for 2 weeks. The liquid is then strained off, and the cucumber bits discarded. This water is very good for closing enlarged pores, and as a skin softener.

Russian Folk Medicine

Complexion milk

The wild tansy (*Tanacetum vulgare*) steeped in buttermilk for nine days, makes the complexion very fair.

Traditional English

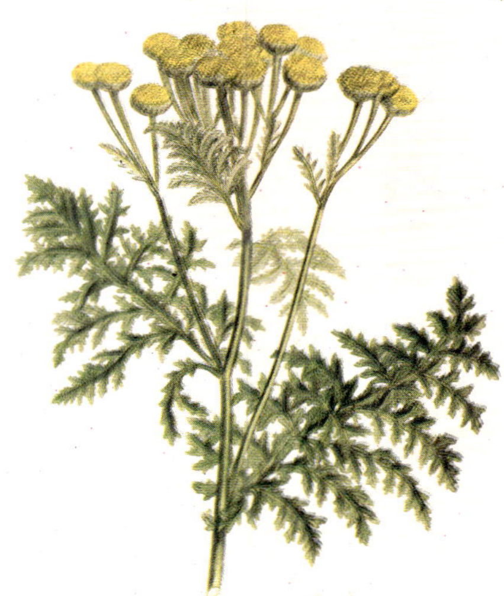

The wild tansy for lovely skin.

FINIS

Fertility and childbirth

Numerous theories existed about conception, and the choice of sex of the infant. All over Europe, and as far away as India, the general belief used to be that semen from the left testicle produced a boy, while that from the right produced a girl. In India, traditionally the wife grabs and squeezes the left testicle to produce a boy; in the 1700's in France, noblemen seeking an heir tied a red silk string tightly round the left one before intercourse.

Among the ancient Hindus, it was believed that priority of orgasm decided the sex of the child. It used to be believed in Scotland that if a girl allowed a man to fondle her during her menstruation, then when she married she could have twins – this is just one of many survivals of menstruation tabus which are found all over the world.

Sterility

Intercourse under a tree was considered good for getting a sterile woman pregnant.

Traditional remedy

In Russia, they used to put willow branches under the bed, with the same idea in mind.

Russian Folk Medicine

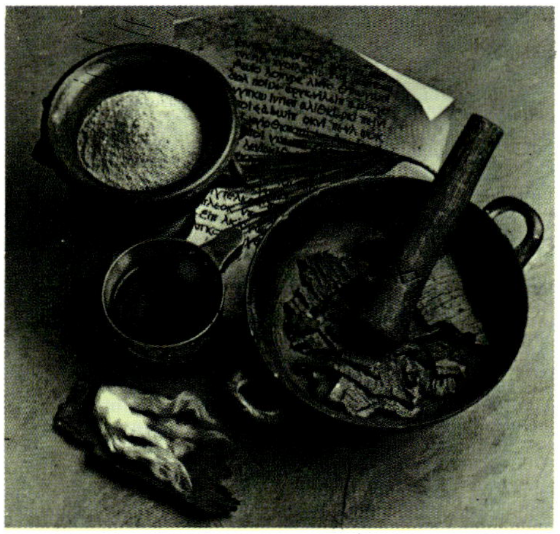

A Greek contraceptive. 'Pine bark, rhus, coriara, both to equal parts: pulverize with wine and use before coitus with the help of wool.'

In Africa, sterility is treated by the folk doctors with plants or fruit bearing evident symbolism – the erect springy stem of a particular flower, or a large unripe banana, for instance.

African Folk Medicine

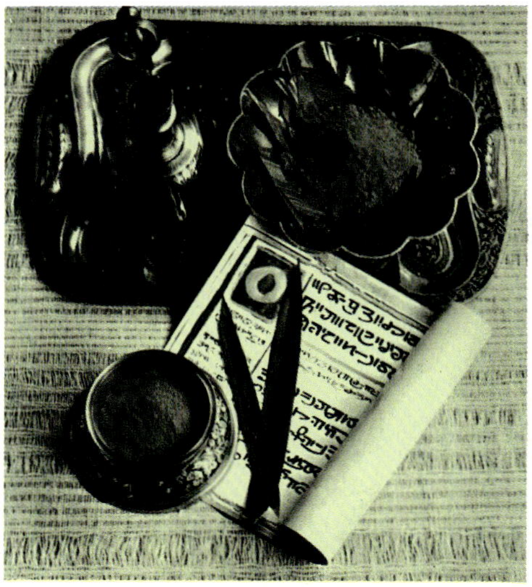

An Indian contraceptive: Palm leaf (powdered) and red chalk taken with cold water on the fourth day of menstruation.

Aphrodisiacs

Ginseng has long been held an aphrodisiac, in Europe, in the Far East, and in North America.

The mandrake is another of folk medicine's oldest aprodisiacs. A special tradition surrounds the procedure of gathering the plant. A dog is tied to the plant, and when he moves he pulls it up. The dog is then killed, otherwise he would go mad. (The importance of this plant is explained by the shape of the root, which vaguely resembles a human body: it was supposed to 'scream' as it was unearthed.)

Impotence

In Northern Europe, horn of a bull used to be recommended for impotence. Spoons made of bull's horn were also considered good for the administering of all medicines.

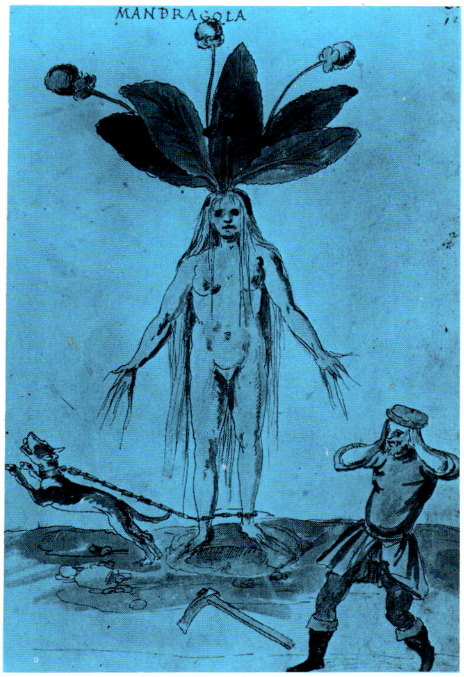

Mandrake, a universal aphrodisiac.

Maternal impression

'Maternal impression' is one of folk medicine's oldest theories, and one that finds a certain degree of acceptance among modern doctors. The basis of the theory is that events occurring to the woman while she carries her baby will be directly transferred to the foetus. The most common variant on this theme in England is the old belief that a woman who sees a hare or puts her foot into a hare's burrow during pregnancy will give birth to a child with a hare lip. This same belief is found among North American Indians.

In German folk lore, a pregnant woman should not enter a courtroom, otherwise her child will be caught up in lifelong litigation. In many primitive societies, women are forbidden to make nets for fishing, or plait ropes, or even plait their hair, for fear of causing a bad birth, or making the umbilical cord strangle the baby. In Scotland it is recorded that women were not supposed to lift their arms to bind up their hair, according to the same principle.

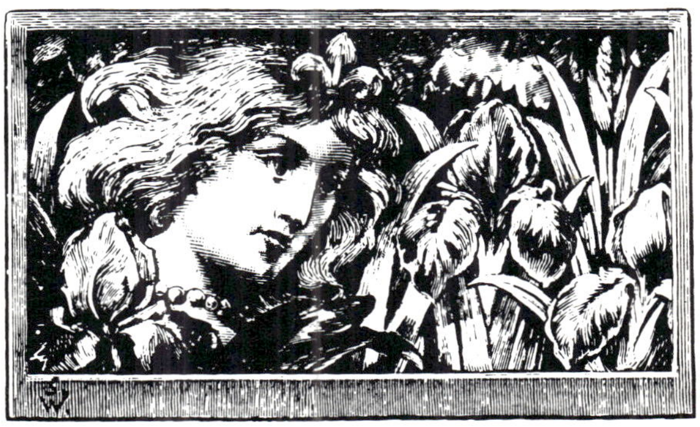

'Only look at beautiful things'

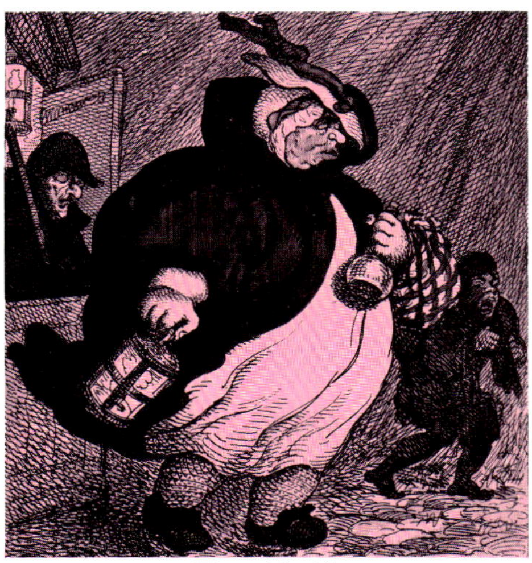

The midwife.

Avoiding tension

The part of this theory that now finds some agreement among modern doctors is that the mother's state of mind may have some bearing on the condition of the baby after its birth: if a mother is especially nervous, tense, or distressed, then the baby is more likely to be difficult. Perhaps pure observation led to the invention of the theory in olden days. One expression of it is the widespread custom for a pregnant woman to avoid going to a funeral. Among many American Indian tribes, expectant women were supposed to look at only beautiful things for their nine months. Some survival of this custom is found in the common notion of a woman having 'whims', especially for tasty or delicate foods during her pregnancy. Perhaps this indulgence, to keep a woman happy, springs from the old folk beliefs.

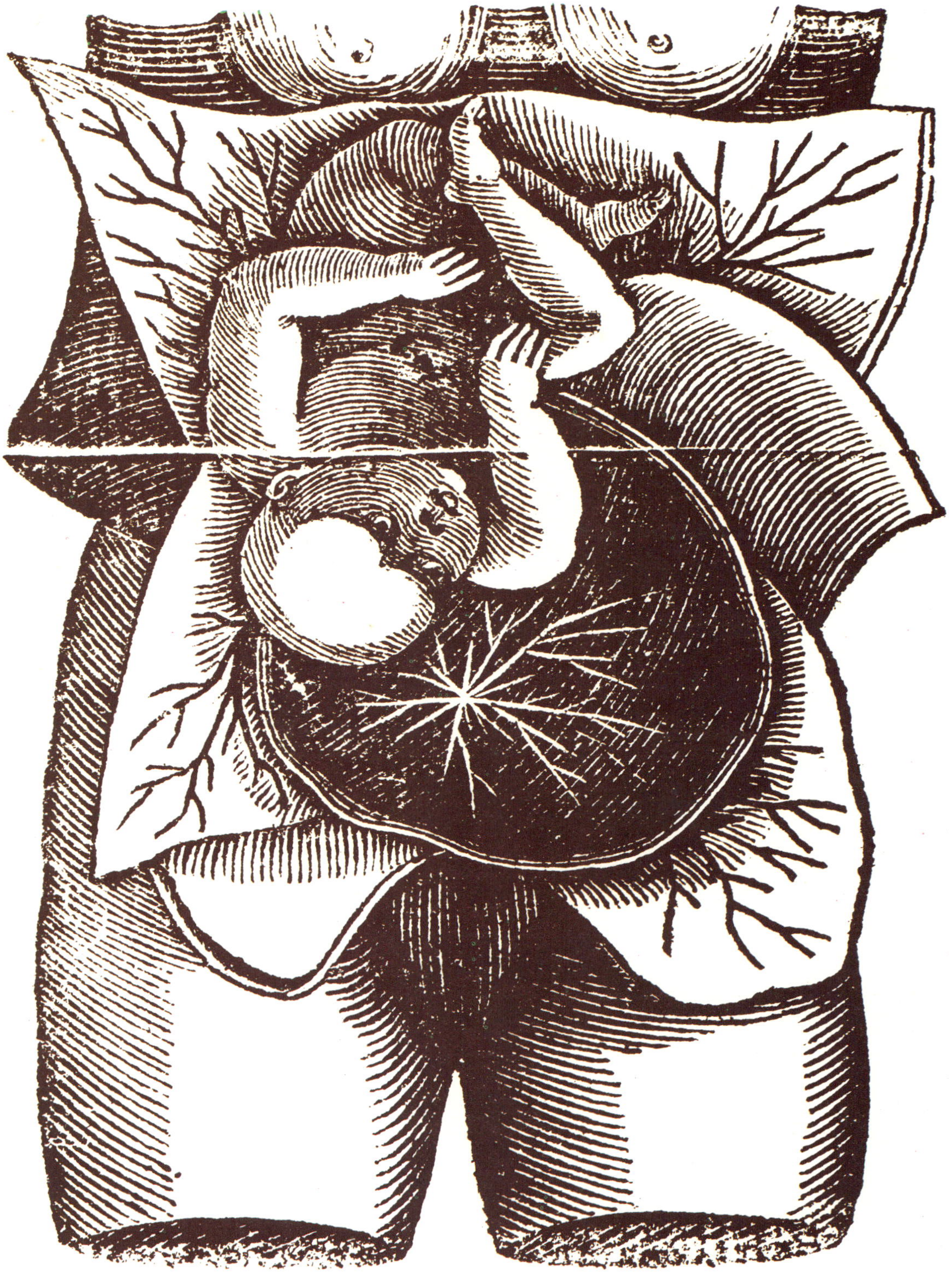

Birth

The actual moment of birth is of such great significance in every society that it is not surprising to find it shrouded in a fog of strange rituals and customs, many of which go beyond the area of folk medicine into religious practice. The curing powers of babies born breech presentation (bottom first) has been mentioned elsewhere. Another lucky sign was to be born with a caul or membrane

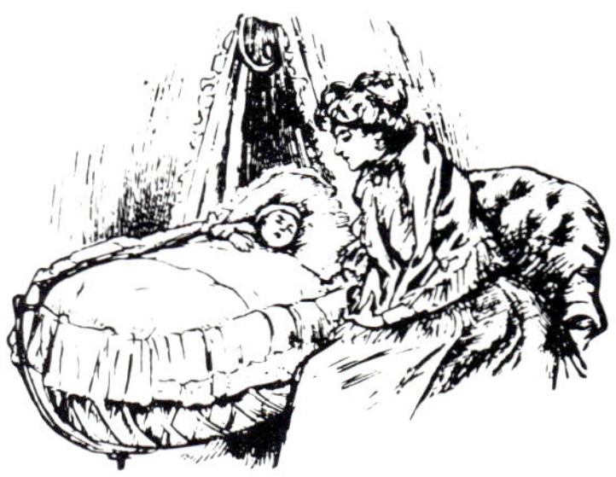

over the head. In France, boy babies born in this way were supposed to be remarkably successful in their love lives. Small bits of the caul were considered to be good luck charms, especially by sailors – a very basic linking up of the idea of birth from the uterine waters with sailing safe into harbour from the sea. Dried placenta has also been imbued with healing powers by many people, notably in China, Java, and other areas of the far east.

Presiding deities

In Jewish mythology, it is Lilith, Adam's love before Eve, who brings bad luck during childbirth. Most societies have some deity who presides over the event, and brings success. In India, it is the elephant-god, Ganesha, god of wisdom. According to the Mohammedan faith at one time, a child born by caesarian section was thought to be the child of the devil, but this seems to be a rare example of negative value attached to this event. Like breech babies, children born by this method are usually considered to be especially blessed, or likely to be remarkable in later life.

This illustration (left) of the birth of a child is from a Victorian edition of Aristotle.

Unbinding customs

Childbirth itself could be eased by 'unlocking' or 'unbinding' customs, found all over the world. Midwives go about the house unlocking bolts and flinging wide the windows. Girdles for wearing

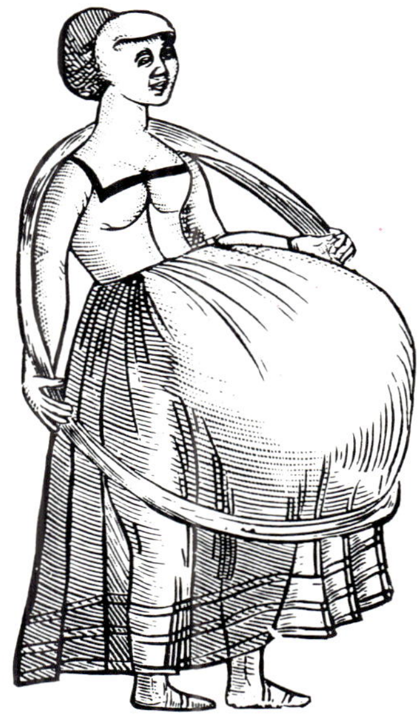

Supporting hoop.

during the labour are found in many parts of the world: in quite recent times, the 1880's, nuns at a convent in Brittany were still making them for presentation to their pupils when they left to get married. In white silk ribbon, the girdle bore the

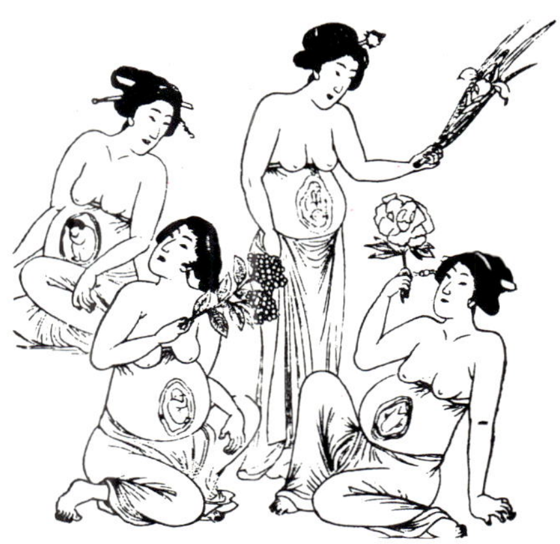

Japanese women wearing tight girdles.

words, 'Notre Dame de Delivrance, protegez-nous.'

In other societies, such as the North American Indian, girdles were worn during the last two months, to prevent the baby rising up so high, presumably with the intention that it would drop and be delivered on time.

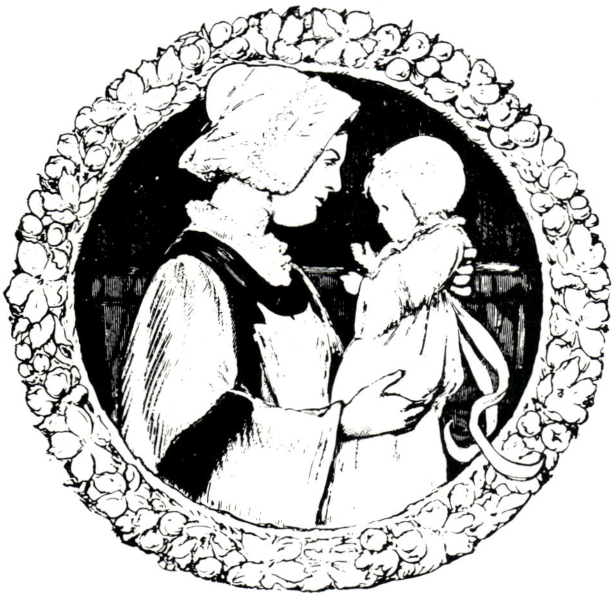

The naevus

Another variation on the maternal impression theory is the idea that events happening to the mother during pregnancy can result in a particular cherry-red mark found on many small children – the *naevus*. (This fades usually within the first year or two). A flower thrown at the mother's face during pregnancy was held to result in this mark in Germany. An old English folk remedy used to be for the mother to lick the naevus with spittle every morning.

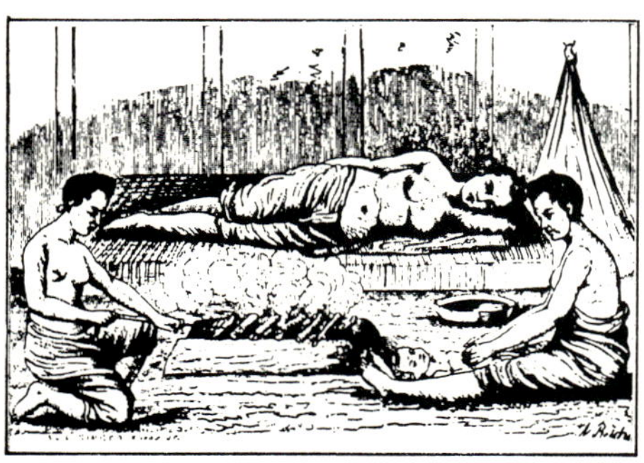

Fumigation was often used to ease delivery of the child.

Drugs for childbirth

To ease labour, ergot has long been used in many parts of the world; another fungus, *ustilago zeae* was used by the Zuni Indians for the same purpose (a substitute tested out by modern medicine). The edible roots of the licorice has been used to help delivery of the placenta in both Europe and North America for several centuries. The Maoris used several aids to facilitate childbirth. The pith of the Nikae (palm) tree was eaten by pregnant women to ease the pelvic muscles, while the sap was drunk to ease labour. The fresh young leaves of the Koromiko shrub were steeped in hot water and given to the mother to promote an easy birth. After delivery, the women would take a steam bath, in which branches of this shrub were used.

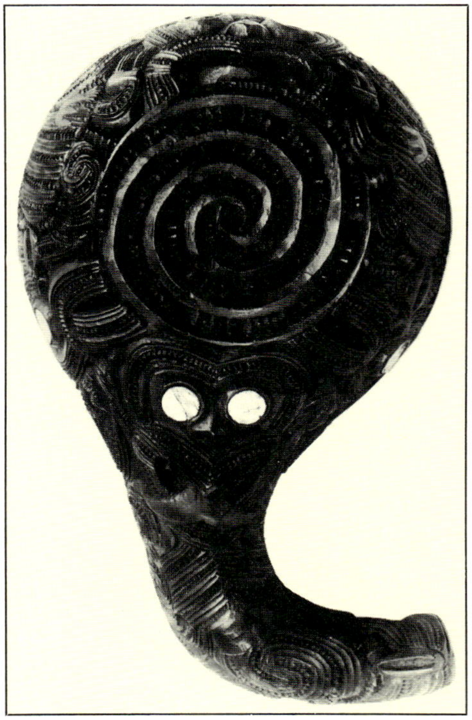

This illustration shows a carved Maori bowl used to receive the afterbirth.

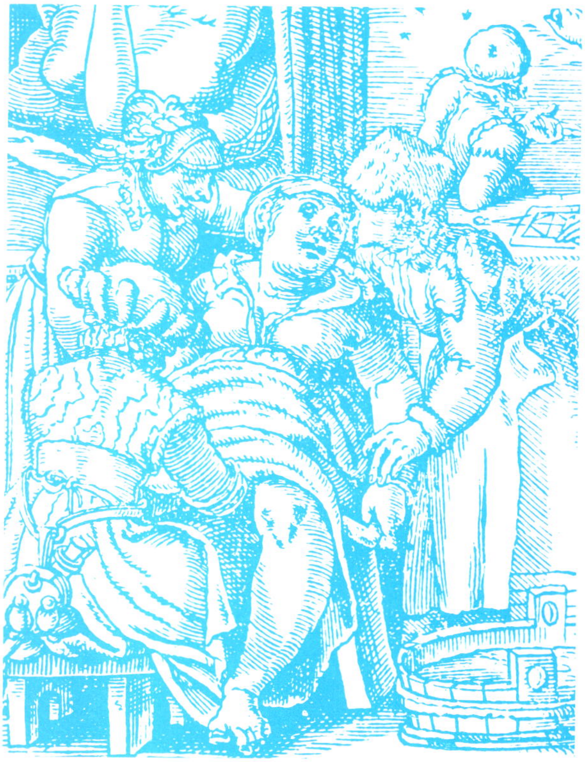

A medieval illustration of a woman in labour.

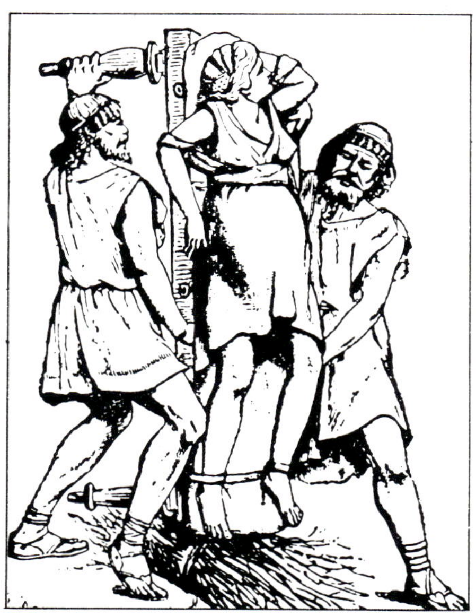

A method of easy delivery. The woman is tied to a couch and up-ended.

Early days after birth

After the birth, every effort was made to make the baby cry or sneeze; until it did so, it was thought to be in the grip of the 'fairies'. In Scotland, an old shoe used to be put on the fire to make bad smoke, and keep off the evil spirits at the birth. Red coral, traditionally used all over Europe for teething rings, is supposed to have the same power, as does silver. (Nowadays we still give silver gifts for a christening, or talk of babies born with silver spoons in their mouths – a sign of good luck.)

Changelings

An unusual story about the power of spirits comes from Scotland, where it used to be thought that some babies were 'changelings' if they cried a good deal. The cure for this was to hold the baby over the fire. If it was a changeling it would shoot up the chimney; a real baby would be protected by the girdle stone (for making oatcakes) that stood always over the flames below. This old superstition led to the phrase, 'If this gangs on we'll need to pit on the girdle'.

Stories about changelings find variations in other continents. In West Africa, a fatalistic version holds that some babies are *abiku*, or born to die, as the result of evil spirits entering the womb. A poem by the modern poet, Wole Soyinka, commemorates the idea:

'In vain your bangles cast
charmed circles at my feet,
I am abiku, calling for the first
And the repeated time.'

Like many other old beliefs, this one is rooted in fact, for it helps to explain away a high infant mortality rate in a primitive society.

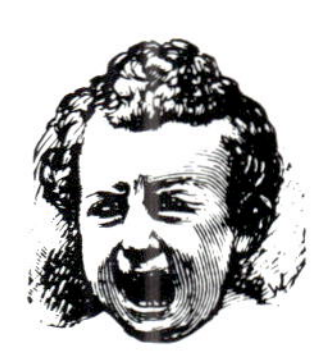

To bring a baby success in life

Once the baby was safely born, yet more customs helped to give it a good start in life. Many surround the navel string: in Australia, aborigines used to put it in water, so that the child would be a strong swimmer. In Mexico, the Indians would bury it in an old battlefield, so that the child would become a brave fighter. The Indians of British Columbia perfected an unusual method of career selection: a piece of the cord would be attached to the ritual mask of a great dancer, so that the baby would become a good dancer in turn, or to the knife of a carver, so that he too would be a craftsman, and so on.

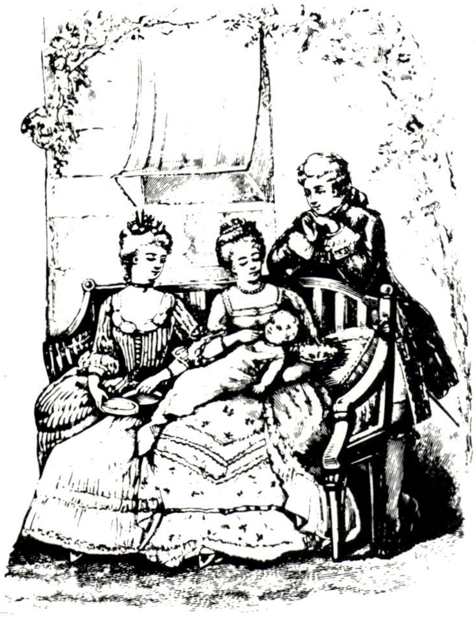

More general wishes for a good future are expressed in the traditional English belief that a baby should always be carried up before he is brought down, so that he will always rise in life, and not fall below his present station. In olden days, midwives went as far as climbing onto a stool rather than bringing the baby downstairs for his first little journey from the birth-bedroom.

It used to be thought bad luck to weigh a baby within the first year of its life, or to cut its finger-nails or hair. In some parts of the world, it is very bad luck to look at a baby upside-down when it is lying in its cradle. Whenever a baby sneezes, it is a good sign, for it means the baby is 'casting out' an evil spirit that is trying to sneak in and take possession. (This explains the still-prevalent custom of saying 'bless you' to someone after a violent sneeze).

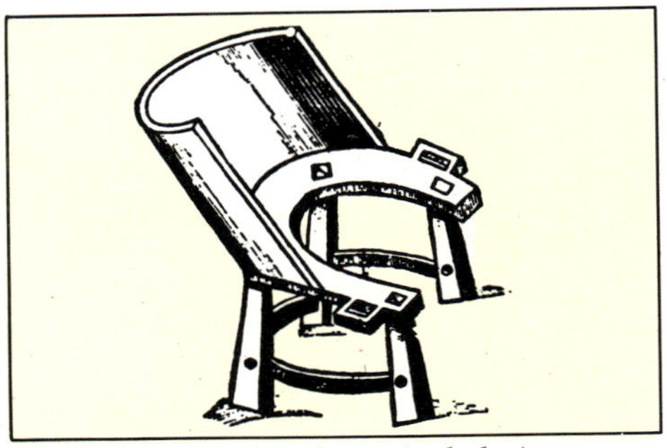

The popular obstetrical chair has been used for centuries.

These are but a handful of the many superstitions, customs, and remedies surrounding pregnancy and birth, but from them it is clearly evident that the moment of birth is but the beginning of a series of significant acts, each of which is imbued with symbolic value, and woven into a framework of comforting, protective explanations.

Nursery rhyme lore

Information about illness and various folk customs for treatment are found in the most surprising places. For example in children's nursery rhymes. One of the most popular is:

Ring-a-ring of roses
A pocket full of posies,
A-tishoo, a-tishoo,
We all fall down.

It is now a widely held theory that this rhyme refers to either the red sores of bubonic plague, or else to a disease called erysipelas, commonly known as St. Anthony's fire, which caused red blotches on the skin like roses. Another, Jack and Jill, has Jill making a poultice of vinegar and brown paper to mend Jack's crown. Vinegar would have been a convenient domestic antiseptic.

The illustration opposite shows Jack and Jill tumbling downhill.

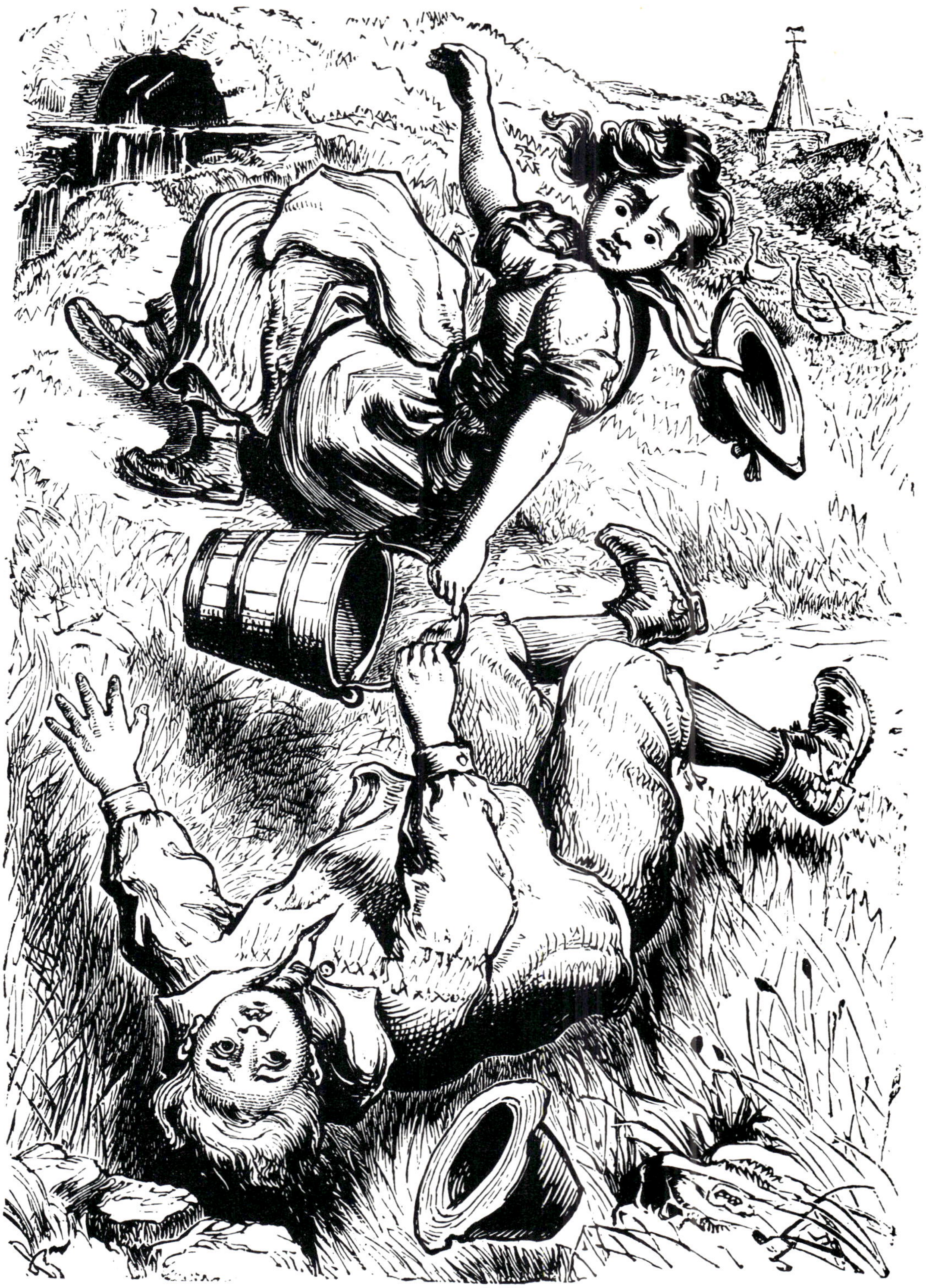

Index for remedies and cures

The following publications are highly recommended for further reading in this area, and have been of invaluable assistance in the preparation of *Folk Medicine: Fact and Fiction.*

Bill Wannan's Australian Folk Medicine
by W. Wannan
William Collins, 1972
Earth Medicine-Earth Foods by Michael Weiner
Macmillan, 1972
Grannie's Remedies by Mai Thomas
Wolfe Publishing, 1965
Magical Medicine by Una Maclean
Allen and Unwin, 1971
Making the Cure by Patrick Logan
Talbot Press, Dublin, 1972
Medicines of the Maori by Christina Macdonald
William Collins, New Zealand, 1974
Russian Folk Medicine by Paul Mark Kourenoff
W. H. Allen, 1972

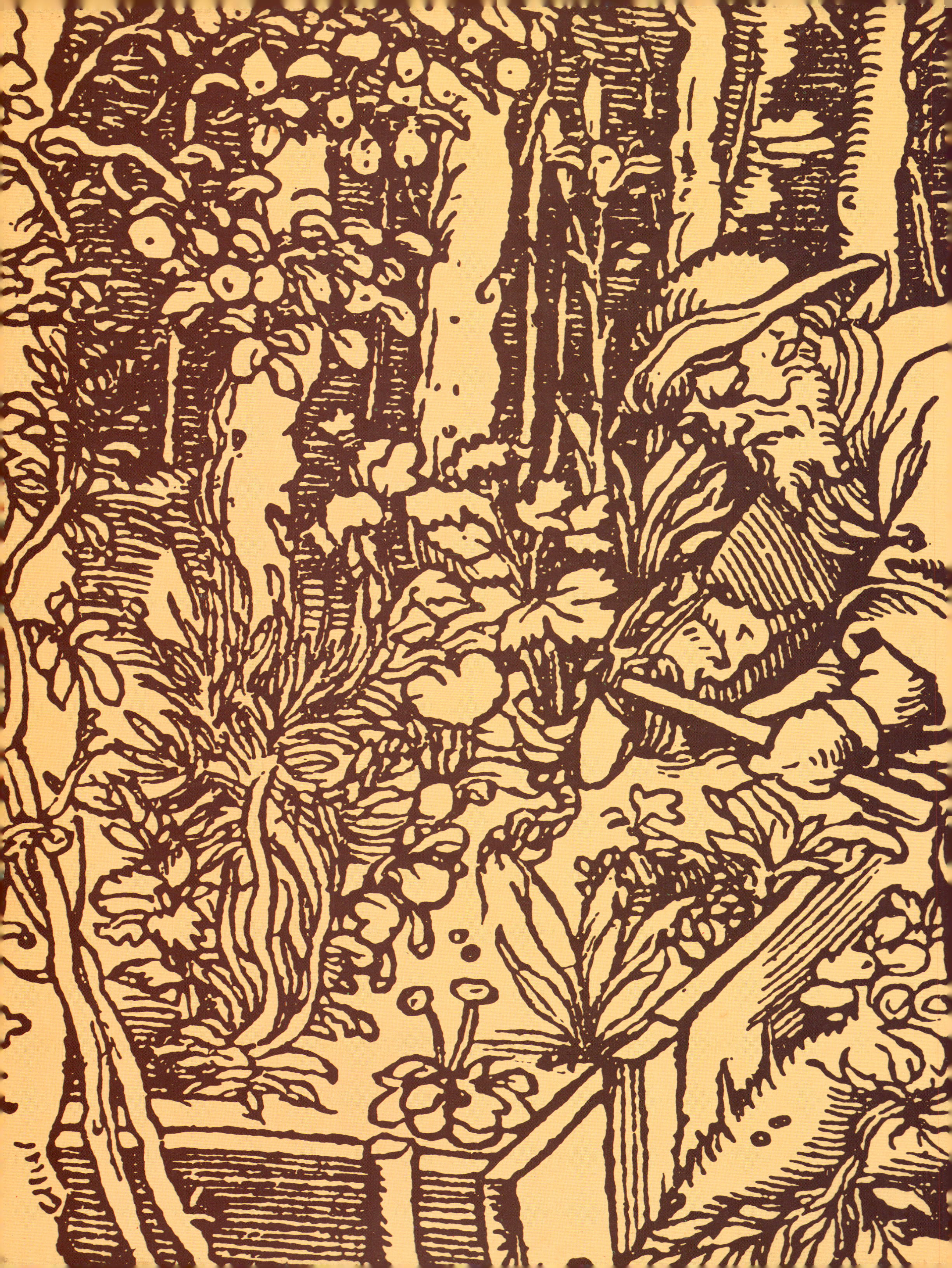